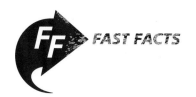

FAST FACTS

3
THIRD
'ON

Bladder Cancer

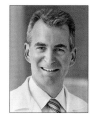

Seth P Lerner MD FACS
Professor, Scott Department of Urology
Beth and Dave Swalm Chair in Urologic Oncology
Director of Urologic Oncology
Director of the Multidisciplinary Bladder Cancer Program
Baylor College of Medicine
Houston, Texas
USA

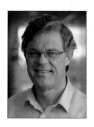

Ian D Davis MB BS (Hons) PhD FRACP FAChPM
Professor of Medicine
Head, Eastern Health Clinical School
Monash University and Eastern Health
Chair, ANZUP Cancer Trials Group
Box Hill, Victoria
Australia

Declaration of Independence
This book is as balanced and as practical a
Ideas for improvement are always welcome: feedb

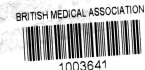

BRITISH MEDICAL ASSOCIATION

1003641

HEALTH PRESS

Fast Facts: Bladder Cancer
First published 1999; second edition 2006
Third edition March 2018

Text © 2018 Seth P. Lerner, Ian D. Davis
© 2018 in this edition Health Press Limited

Health Press Limited, Elizabeth House, Queen Street, Abingdon,
Oxford OX14 3LN, UK. Tel: +44 (0)1235 523233

Book orders can be placed by telephone or via the website.
For regional distributors or to order via the website, please go to:
www.fastfacts.com. For telephone orders, please call 01752 202301

Fast Facts is a trademark of Health Press Limited.

A CIP record for this title is available from the British Library.

ISBN 978-1-910797-64-8

Lerner SP (Seth P)
Fast Facts: Bladder Cancer/
Seth P. Lerner, Ian D. Davis

Medical illustrations by Dee McLean and Graeme Chambers.
Typesetting by Thomas Bohm, User Design, Illustration and Typesetting, UK.
Printed in the UK with Xpedient Print.

IDD is supported by an NHMRC Practitioner Fellowship (APP1102604).

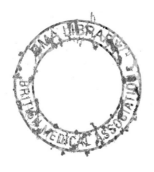

Glossary

BCG: bacillus Calmette–Guérin

BTA: bladder tumor antigen

CI: confidence interval

CIS: carcinoma in situ

CMV: cisplatin–methotrexate–vinblastine

CT: computed tomography

CTLA-4: cytotoxic T-lymphocyte-associated protein 4

CTU: computed tomographic urography

ECOG: Eastern Cooperative Oncology Group

ERAS: Enhanced Recovery After Surgery (protocol)

FDA: US Food and Drug Administration

FGFR: fibroblast growth factor receptor

GC: gemcitabine + cisplatin chemotherapy

GFR: glomerular filtration rate

HER2: human epidermal growth factor receptor 2

HG: high-grade

MIBC: muscle-invasive bladder cancer

MRI: magnetic resonance imaging

MVAC: methotrexate–vinblastine–doxorubicin–cisplatin

NMIBC: non-muscle-invasive bladder cancer

OS: overall survival

PD-1: programmed cell death protein 1

PD-L1: programmed cell death ligand 1

PS: performance status

TCGA: The Cancer Genome Atlas

TNM: tumor–nodes–metastases (staging system)

TURBT: transurethral resection of bladder tumor

UC: urothelial cancer

UTI: urinary tract infection

VEGFR: vascular endothelial growth factor receptor

WHO: World Health Organization

Introduction

Bladder cancer accounts for significant cancer-related morbidity, mortality and healthcare expenditure in most parts of the world. The management of low-grade non-muscle-invasive bladder cancer has changed little in recent times, although surgical technology and techniques continue to improve. Intravesical immunotherapy with bacillus Calmette–Guérin (BCG) remains the standard of care for high-grade non-muscle-invasive disease. Initial response rates are high with BCG but disease recurrence is common, and the risk of progression to muscle-invasive cancer increases with time since the first BCG treatment.

Recent years have seen rapid advances in our understanding of the biology of bladder cancer, including the identification of molecular subtypes that are clinically significant. Perioperative systemic cytotoxic chemotherapy for localized muscle-invasive bladder cancer has now been widely adopted, although rates of use vary. Chemotherapy is still frequently used for advanced or metastatic bladder cancer. The most promising recent advance has been the development of immunotherapy approaches that target the programmed cell death protein 1 (PD-1) axis and other immune checkpoints; five immunotherapies that target the PD-1 axis have recently been approved for use in advanced urothelial cancer, and numerous clinical trials are in progress across all stages of the disease and lines of treatment. Whilst these new treatments offer hope to patients, for clinicians there is a lot to understand in terms of how these immunotherapies are best used: who they are suitable for, the point at which each treatment should be used, and the sequencing of treatments for individual patients.

Fast Facts: Bladder Cancer provides a concise guide to help clinicians and patients understand the evidence underlying various treatment options and approaches; it is not intended to be either exhaustive or exhausting. This third edition has been updated throughout, with significant updates to the chapter on pathology and biology, including discussion of new molecular targets; it also includes a new chapter about immunotherapy for bladder cancer. Our thanks go to Derek Raghavan and Michael Bailey for their work on the previous editions. We hope that you find *Fast Facts: Bladder Cancer* to be a helpful resource.

1 Epidemiology and etiology

Epidemiology

An estimated 541 000 new cases of bladder cancer occurred globally in 2016, with 188 000 deaths.[1] In the UK, approximately 10 100 new cases were diagnosed in 2014, accounting for 3% of all new cancer cases; bladder cancer is the tenth most common cancer in the UK.[2] The estimated annual incidence of bladder cancer in the USA in 2018 is expected to be 81 190, with 17 240 deaths.[3]

Bladder cancer is more common in men than women, with a male-to-female incidence ratio of 4:1, although the incidence among women appears to be rising.[1] The global age-standardized incidence is 14.1 per 100 000 person-years for men and 3.6 for women.[1] Bladder cancer is the fourth most common cancer in men in the USA. Incidence increases with age, with a median age at presentation of over 75 years in the UK.[3]

Most cases of bladder cancer are non-muscle-invasive urothelial cancers, which can usually be cured; the 5-year survival rate for these cancers is more than 95%. However, invasive or metastatic bladder cancer is a frequent cause of cancer death, accounting for approximately 17 000 deaths annually in the USA and 188 000 globally.[3] Age-standardized death rates for bladder cancer are 5.1 per 100 000 person-years in men and 1.5 per 100 000 person-years in women.[1] Survival rates at different stages of the disease are reported on page 25. Globally, bladder cancer is responsible for over 3 million disability-adjusted life-years, mainly years of life lost due to advanced disease.[1]

Some data suggest that the global impact of bladder cancer is decreasing, even though incidence continues to rise, with a 9.6% decrease in the age-standardized rate for years of life lost between 2005 and 2015.[1] Other data suggest that survival may be decreasing, although these findings may reflect differences in coding or age at diagnosis.[4] Variable access to healthcare is likely to play a significant role.

All stages of presentation are more common in Africa, the Middle East, Central America, and Asia, and less common in affluent countries. The lifetime risk of developing bladder cancer before 79 years of age is 1/36 for men and 1/165 for women in high sociodemographic index countries, and 1/122 and 1/310, respectively, in low sociodemographic index countries.

Etiology

Numerous factors are implicated in bladder carcinogenesis, as shown in Table 1.1. These include host factors (e.g. age, sex, comorbidities, familial cancer syndromes), social and economic influences and

TABLE 1.1

Factors implicated in the etiology of bladder cancer

Host factors
- Sex
- Age
- Ethnicity
- Chronic urinary tract infection
- Bladder stones
- Congenital bladder defects
- Familial cancer syndromes:
  - *PTEN* (Cowden syndrome)
  - DNA mismatch repair genes such as *MLH1*, *MSH2*, *MSH6* and *PMS2* (Lynch syndrome or hereditary nonpolyposis colon cancer syndrome)
  - *RB1* (retinoblastoma syndrome)
- Other mutations: *GNT*, *NAT*
- Single-nucleotide polymorphisms:
  - *MTHFD2* (methyl metabolism)
  - *TEP1* (telomerase)
  - Decreased risk with *IL8RB*
  - Shorter survival with *CASP9*
  - Longer survival with low activity of *EPHX1* gene (metabolizes carcinogens)

CONTINUED

TABLE 1.1 (CONTINUED)

Factors implicated in the etiology of bladder cancer

Social and economic factors	• Geographic location • Sociodemographic index
Environmental or occupational exposure	• Tobacco smoking (including secondary or sidestream/passive exposure to tobacco smoke) • 2-Naphthylamine • 4-Aminobiphenyl • Aniline dyes • Arsenic • Benzidine • Benzo[a]pyrene • Beta-naphthylamine • Chlornaphazine • Dichlorobenzidine • Diesel exhaust • 4,4'-methylene-bis-ortho-chloroaniline (MOCA) • Ortho-dianisidine • Ortho-toluidine • Phenacetin
Iatrogenic (medical) exposure	• Cyclophosphamide • Diagnostic and therapeutic radiation

exposure to carcinogens. Many of these are avoidable, and as a result, many cases of bladder cancer could be prevented. The importance of genetic factors is discussed in more detail on page 21.

Smoking. Cigarette smoking is a major contributor to bladder carcinogenesis: 60–80% of patients with bladder cancer have a history of cigarette smoking and smoking increases the risk of bladder cancer by 2–5-fold.[5] Smokers also have a higher rate of tumor recurrence than non-smokers, and a greater proportion of tumors of higher stage and grade.

Sidestream (secondary/passive) exposure to cigarette smoke is also a significant but insidious risk factor that may be difficult to avoid. This risk is particularly increased in individuals who have cytochrome P450 CYP1A2 fast metabolizer or *N*-acetyltransferase-2 slow-acetylation phenotypes.[6]

Cigar and pipe tobacco smoking are also associated with an increased risk of bladder cancer, although the effect size seems to be less than with cigarettes.[7]

The role of 'vaping' with e-cigarettes or similar devices is unclear. Animal studies have demonstrated the presence of DNA adducts and inhibition of DNA repair, and several small studies have demonstrated the presence of known carcinogens in the urine of vapers, such as 2-naphthylamine and ortho-toluidine.[8]

No clear increase in the risk of bladder cancer has been reported in marijuana smokers. One cohort study suggested an inverse association, although a causal effect has not been established.[9]

Occupational risks. The strongest association between occupation and bladder cancer has been identified in workers of aniline dyes who are exposed to aromatic amines. Other occupations associated with an increased risk of bladder cancer due to carcinogen exposure are listed in Table 1.2. Occupational risks have been reviewed by Rushton et al.[10] and Burger et al.[11]

Dietary factors. The importance of dietary factors in the etiology of bladder cancer remains unclear. Most studies have been cohort or case–control studies and have not included detailed dietary information. Caffeine has long been thought to be implicated in bladder cancer but the effects of confounding factors have been difficult to untangle. A meta-analysis of case–control and cohort studies concluded that coffee consumption was associated with a 33% increase in the odds ratio for development of bladder cancer,[12] and the argument was strengthened by the finding that bladder cancer risk was increased in non-smoking coffee drinkers. Overall, the relationship has been hard to define because of the widespread use of caffeine and its association with other known carcinogens such as those associated with smoking. Current consensus is that normal doses of caffeine are not bladder carcinogenic.

TABLE 1.2

Industries associated with exposure to bladder carcinogens

Aluminum smelting

Dye manufacture

Hairdressing and hair dyes

Leather workers

Painting

Pest control

Petroleum refining and petrochemical manufacture

Printing

Production of coal gas

Rubber manufacture (especially tires and cables)

Sewage work

Textile printing

Truck driving (diesel)

Various artificial sweeteners have been implicated as risk factors for bladder cancer but subsequent research has failed to confirm such links; the US Food and Drug Administration does not list any restrictions for artificial sweeteners with respect to bladder cancer risk.

Long-term ingestion of drinking water contaminated with nitrate derived from fertilizers or human or animal waste has been linked with an increased risk of bladder cancer in postmenopausal women.[13]

Cyclophosphamide, used in the treatment of various malignancies and autoimmune conditions, sometimes at very high doses, has known bladder carcinogenic effects.[14] A dose–response relationship is evident: cumulative doses above 20 g increase the risk 6-fold, and doses of 50 g or more increase the risk by 14.5-fold. Latency is relatively short – the time between exposure and subsequent bladder cancer diagnosis is 6–13 years. The risk of subsequent bladder cancer can be reduced in the oncology setting by minimizing the cumulative dose, although this is not always feasible. Co-administration of the chemoprotectant 2-mercaptoethanesulfonic acid (MESNA) reduces the rate of cyclophosphamide-related cystitis and may reduce the risk of subsequent bladder cancer.[15]

Pelvic irradiation for conditions such as cervical cancer has been linked to a 4-fold increase in the risk of bladder cancer.[11] Although modern radiation therapy techniques aim to spare the bladder and other structures, these organs are nevertheless exposed to significant doses of radiation and it is impossible to completely avoid a risk of subsequent new primary cancers at these sites.

Chronic infection or inflammation due to indwelling suprapubic or Foley catheters in patients with spinal cord injury and other conditions has been linked to an increased incidence of bladder cancer, especially squamous cell cancer.[11] Chronic kidney stones may also lead to chronic inflammation and an increased risk of bladder cancer.

Schistosomiasis (also known as snail fever and bilharzia) due to *Schistosoma haematobium* is the most common cause of bladder cancer in some areas of Egypt; the incidence can be as high as 70%. Most bladder cancers related to schistosomiasis have squamous cell histology although urothelial cancers also occur.

Key points – epidemiology and etiology

- Bladder cancer is a common tumor; each year approximately 17 000 people in the USA die from the disease, and 188 000 globally.
- Bladder cancer incidence has a male-to-female ratio of 4:1. The incidence increases with age, with a median age at presentation of 60–65 years.
- Bladder cancer has many etiological risk factors, most of which are avoidable; the most common cause is cigarette smoking.
- Some familial syndromes and genetic predispositions increase the risk of bladder cancer.

Key references

1. Global Burden of Disease Cancer Collaboration. Global, regional, and national cancer incidence, mortality, years of life lost, years lived with disability, and disability-adjusted life-years for 32 cancer groups, 1990 to 2015: A systematic analysis for the global burden of disease study. *JAMA Oncol* 2017;3:524–48.

2. Cancer Research UK. *Bladder cancer statistics*. 2017. www.cancerresearchuk.org/health-professional/cancer-statistics/statistics-by-cancer-type/bladder-cancer.

3. Siegel RL, Miller KD, Jemal A. Cancer statistics, 2018. *CA Cancer J Clin* 2018;68:7–30.

4. Australian Institute of Health and Welfare. Cancer survival and prevalence in Australia: Period estimates from 1982 to 2010. *Asia Pac J Clin Oncol* 2013;9:29–39.

5. Rink M, Crivelli JJ, Shariat SF et al. Smoking and bladder cancer: a systematic review of risk and outcomes. *Eur Urol Focus* 2015;1:17–27.

6. Tao L, Xiang YB, Wang R et al. Environmental tobacco smoke in relation to bladder cancer risk – the Shanghai bladder cancer study [corrected]. *Cancer Epidemiol Biomarkers Prev* 2010;19:3087–95.

7. Pitard A, Brennan P, Clavel J et al. Cigar, pipe, and cigarette smoking and bladder cancer risk in European men. *Cancer Causes Control* 2001;12:551–6.

8. Fuller T, Acharya A, Bhaskar G et al. MP88-14 Evaluation of e-cigarettes users urine for known bladder carcinogens. *J Urol* 2017;197:e1179.

9. Thomas AA, Wallner LP, Quinn VP et al. Association between cannabis use and the risk of bladder cancer: results from the California Men's Health Study. *Urology* 2015;85:388–92.

10. Rushton L, Bagga S, Bevan R et al. Occupation and cancer in Britain. *Br J Cancer* 2010;102:1428–37.

11. Burger M, Catto JW, Dalbagni G et al. Epidemiology and risk factors of urothelial bladder cancer. *Eur Urol* 2013;63:234–41.

12. Wu W, Tong Y, Zhao Q et al. Coffee consumption and bladder cancer: a meta-analysis of observational studies. *Sci Rep* 2015;5:9051.

13. Jones RR, Weyer PJ, DellaValle CT et al. Nitrate from drinking water and diet and bladder cancer among postmenopausal women in Iowa. *Environ Health Perspect* 2016;124:1751–8.

14. Travis LB, Curtis RE, Glimelius B et al. Bladder and kidney cancer following cyclophosphamide therapy for non-Hodgkin's lymphoma. *J Natl Cancer Inst* 1995;87:524–30.

15. Monach PA, Arnold LM, Merkel PA. Incidence and prevention of bladder toxicity from cyclophosphamide in the treatment of rheumatic diseases: a data-driven review. *Arthritis Rheum* 2010;62:9–21.

Pathology and biology

Histology

The histological types of primary carcinoma that occur in the bladder are shown in Table 2.1.

Urothelial cancer (UC; Figure 2.1) is derived from the transitional epithelium. It accounts for almost 90% of the bladder cancers that occur in industrialized countries such as the USA and the UK, and most discussion of bladder cancer relates to this type. Such tumors may be papillary (confined to the urothelium or lamina propria) (70–75%) or solid and invasive (20–25%).[1]

TABLE 2.1

Histological types of primary cancers that occur in the bladder

- Urothelial (formerly 'transitional cell cancer') – may be pure or mixed with histological variants
  - Papillary and exophytic (Ta) – may be confined to epithelium or invasive into lamina propria; papillary morphology may also be seen in muscle-invasive cancer
  - Solid and invasive
  - Carcinoma in situ (CIS, also known as Tis)
- Squamous cell carcinoma
- Adenocarcinoma
- Micropapillary
- Small-cell neuroendocrine cancer
- Sarcomatoid
- Lymphoepithelial-like
- Plasmacytoid
- Nested

Carcinoma in situ (CIS) is an additional and important type seen in about 10% of cases (sometimes as secondary CIS associated with papillary UC). CIS is a flat, intraepithelial, high-grade carcinoma, often with increased numbers of mitotic structures. In approximately half of all cases, CIS occurs as one or more de novo lesions (primary CIS), while in the remainder it occurs in association with either papillary or solid tumors (secondary CIS). Coexistent CIS and papillary non-muscle-invasive bladder cancer confers a worse prognosis than papillary disease alone.

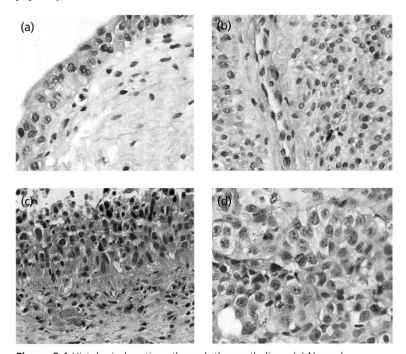

Figure 2.1 Histological sections through the urothelium. (a) Normal urothelium, which is 3–7 cells thick and lies between the basement membrane and an intact layer of umbrella cells on the luminal surface. (b) In low-grade papillary urothelial carcinoma, the urothelial cells have a slightly increased nucleus-to-cytoplasm ratio, and umbrella cells are lost. A fibrovascular stalk is usually prominent. (c) Carcinoma in situ is a high-grade intraepithelial cancer. (d) High-grade urothelial carcinoma is characterized by a wide range of cell shapes and sizes. The nucleus-to-cytoplasm ratio is very high, mitoses are occasional to frequent, and many cells have multiple nucleoli.

UC can coexist with elements of squamous and glandular differentiation. The classification of the tumor depends on the dominant histological type.

An important development has been the identification of a common stem cell of origin in xenograft and cell culture studies. This stem cell type has features of UC as well as showing squamous and glandular differentiation within individual tumor cells. This may explain why metastases with variant histology (e.g. as squamous cell carcinoma or adenocarcinoma) are seen in patients with pure UC primary tumors.

Squamous cell carcinoma has a nodular, infiltrative growth pattern and is usually invasive. It accounts for 5–10% of bladder cancers in the USA and UK. Historically, squamous cell carcinoma accounted for up to 70% of bladder cancers in areas where schistosomiasis is endemic, such as Egypt (see page 12), whereas contemporary data suggest that UC is now the predominant histology in Egypt as the prevalence of schistosomiasis has decreased.[2] Squamous cell carcinoma is also associated with chronic infection or inflammation, such as that due to indwelling suprapubic catheters.[3]

Adenocarcinoma is rare, accounting for about 2% of bladder cancers. Approximately 30–35% of adenocarcinomas are derived from the urachus and classically appear as a solid, invasive-appearing tumor in the dome of the bladder. (The urachus is the remnant of the embryonic cavity, the allantois; it usually forms a fibrous cord connecting the bladder to the umbilicus.) The remainder of adenocarcinomas are associated with bladder exstrophy or are non-urachal in origin.

Adenocarcinomas are usually solitary, high grade and ulcerative. They can be difficult to distinguish histologically from adenocarcinomas of the colon or rectum, and clinical determination of the source is often difficult. Any bladder adenocarcinoma may be mucin-producing. Many patients with adenocarcinoma have poor prognosis because the tumor is already at an advanced stage at diagnosis. Urachal adenocarcinomas present as invasive tumors often visible on the dome of the bladder and tend to be asymptomatic until late in the disease course, since they arise in a minimally functional part of the bladder. Surgical therapy is closed partial cystectomy.[4]

Micropapillary cancer (Figure 2.2) is a particularly aggressive form of high-grade UC and is associated with a high risk of early muscle invasion and metastasis. Lymphovascular invasion is seen in more than 50% of cases. Amplification of human *Her2* and/or increased HER2 protein expression has been reported with this variant[5] and the proportion of the tumor that is micropapillary may correlate with outcome.

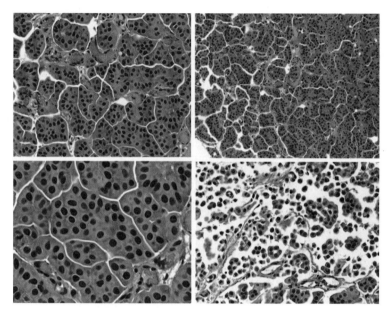

Figure 2.2 Micropapillary cancer is a variant of high-grade urothelial cancer. Each panel reflects variations in morphology.

Small-cell neuroendocrine bladder cancer is similar to the more common small-cell cancer of the lung. This histological pattern is associated with rapid growth and early metastasis, and may occur as a pure variant or mixed with typical UC. These tumors typically stain positive for chromogranin A (which can also be measured in the peripheral blood) and synaptophysin (Figure 2.3). The cells have a high nucleus-to-cytoplasm ratio, and grow in sheets or nests of cells. This variant should be distinguished from undifferentiated UC, which is the least differentiated of the UCs.

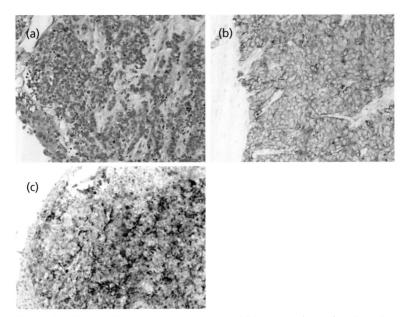

Figure 2.3 Small-cell neuroendocrine cancer. (a) Hematoxylin and eosin stain; (b) synaptophysin stain; (c) chromogranin stain.

Sarcomatoid bladder cancer is a rare variant, accounting for 0.3% of cases. It contains morphologic features of epithelial elements expressing cytokeratin (which may be urothelial, squamous, neuroendocrine or adenocarcinoma) and malignant mesenchymal 'sarcoma' elements (leiomyosarcoma, chondrosarcoma, rhabdomyosarcoma, liposarcoma). It may be associated with past exposure to cyclophosphamide or radiation.

Lymphoepithelial-like bladder cancer accounts for 0.4–1.3% of bladder cancers. Morphologically, it resembles nasopharyngeal lymphoepithelioma, with syncytial sheets of undifferentiated tumor cells with minimal cytoplasm, prominent nucleoli, many mitoses and the presence of lymphocytes and reactive cells, including histiocytes, eosinophils and plasma cells. It does not stain for Epstein–Barr virus markers, distinguishing it from certain lymphomas. Immunohistochemical diagnosis includes identification of both lymphocyte and epithelial cell markers.

Plasmacytoid urothelial cancer, as the name suggests, resembles lymphoma or plasmacytoma. About 3% of bladder cancers contain this variant.[6] Immunohistochemistry demonstrates expression of epithelial markers such as cytokeratins or epithelial membrane antigen, and plasma cell markers such as CD138. Expression of GATA3 can be useful to distinguish these lesions from plasmacytomas, particularly in the metastatic setting when the epithelial component might be missed.

Nested variant urothelial cancer is also rare, accounting for 0.3% of invasive cancers. It can be aggressive despite a relatively innocuous cellular morphology. Cells are usually only mildly atypical, although the deep interface with the stroma may show irregularity and infiltration, with more atypical cellular features at greater depth and evidence of retraction artifact. Nested variant is not associated with overlying CIS, and cannot be classified as high grade.

'Field changes' of a probable premalignant nature are often found in association with bladder cancer, and range from atypia to mild or severe dysplasia. The term refers to the concept that the entire tissue is abnormal at some genetic level, even if there is no macroscopic evidence of disease. The recognition of such changes is important in determining the risk of recurrence and progression. Normal transitional epithelium has a superficial layer of large, flat umbrella cells, beneath which are 3–7 layers of regular cells (Figure 2.1a). These lie above a basement membrane that separates the mucosa from the underlying lamina propria. The World Health Organization (WHO) has recently reclassified urothelial neoplasms and recognizes hyperplasia as well as four types of atypia.[7] These include dysplasia (low-grade intraurothelial neoplasia) and CIS (high-grade intraurothelial neoplasia, formerly classified as severe dysplasia). Atypia indicates the presence of an increased number of cell layers, with loss of polarity of a still-intact umbrella layer. Dysplasia refers to an increase in the size of nuclei that are basally located and exhibit loss of polarity but the cell layers are not increased in number.

Staging and grading

Accurate staging and grading of UC is essential, as it determines the most effective treatment. Understaging and undergrading may lead to inappropriate decisions about primary treatment modalities or perioperative systemic chemotherapy, increasing the risk of adverse outcomes for the patient.

Staging. The tumor–nodes–metastases (TNM) staging of the American Joint Committee on Cancer is the system most widely used for bladder cancer, illustrated in Figures 2.4 and 2.5.

The seventh edition of the TNM staging (introduced in January 2010[8]) was replaced by the eighth edition from 1 January 2018 (available from cancerstaging.org). The only material change in the staging of bladder cancer is the addition of invasion of seminal vesicles to the T4a stage.

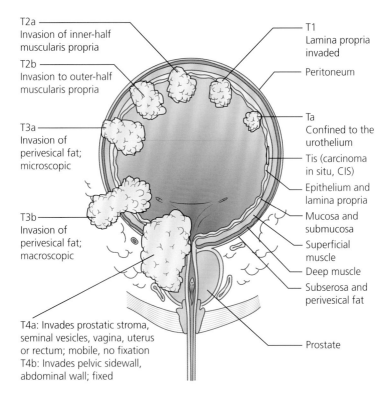

T2a
Invasion of inner-half muscularis propria

T2b
Invasion to outer-half muscularis propria

T3a
Invasion of perivesical fat; microscopic

T3b
Invasion of perivesical fat; macroscopic

T4a: Invades prostatic stroma, seminal vesicles, vagina, uterus or rectum; mobile, no fixation
T4b: Invades pelvic sidewall, abdominal wall; fixed

T1
Lamina propria invaded

Peritoneum

Ta
Confined to the urothelium

Tis (carcinoma in situ, CIS)

Epithelium and lamina propria

Mucosa and submucosa

Superficial muscle

Deep muscle

Subserosa and perivesical fat

Prostate

Figure 2.4 Tumor staging of bladder cancer according to the 2018 American Joint Committee on Cancer Staging Manual. The tumor stage is determined from the level of invasion into or through the bladder wall and invasion of adjacent organs.

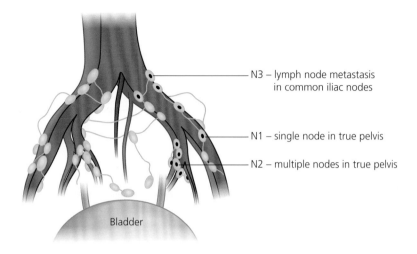

Figure 2.5 Current node staging system for bladder cancer, as per the eighth edition of the tumor–node–metastasis staging system. The true (or lesser) pelvis refers to the space enclosed by the pelvic girdle and below the pelvic brim, between the pelvic inlet and the pelvic floor. It includes the external and internal, obturator and presacral nodes. At least 12 nodes must be evaluated for adequate staging.

Grading. The current grading system, introduced in 2004, stratifies bladder cancer into low and high grade, replacing the WHO 1973 three-grade system[7], as illustrated in Figure 2.6. Approximately 40% of former grade 2 tumors are reclassified as high grade in the current system, and grade 1 tumors are stratified into papillary urothelial neoplasm of low malignant potential or low-grade cancers. Many pathologists will report according to both systems when a high-grade cancer has features of former grade 2, in order to give the treating physician greater understanding of the potential behavior of a particular cancer (Figure 2.6).

Molecular phenotype

Genomic profiling of non-muscle-invasive and muscle-invasive bladder cancer reveals substantial molecular diversity, suggesting that bladder cancer comprises multiple genomic phenotypes, reflecting the clinical and histological heterogeneity. Low-grade tumors are characterized by a high frequency of *FGFR3* mutations, 9q loss of heterozygosity and

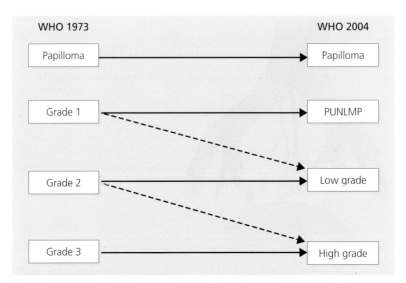

Figure 2.6 Relationship between the 1973 and current 2004 World Health Organization (WHO) grading systems for urothelial bladder cancer. Pathologists may report using both systems to provide more detailed information about the likely behavior of a particular tumor. PUNLMP, papillary urothelial neoplasm of low malignant potential.

alterations in *PIK3CA* and *STAG2*.[9] High-grade cancers have frequent cell cycle alterations, with mutations in *p53* and *RB1* and 9p and 9q loss of heterozygosity.[9] The Cancer Genome Atlas (TCGA) project recently reported comprehensive integrated genomic analysis of 412 muscle-invasive cancers.[10] These cancers were characterized by a high somatic mutation rate, similar to that in lung cancer and melanoma, with 58 significantly mutated genes. The high mutation load was associated with APOBEC (apolipoprotein B mRNA editing enzyme, catalytic polypeptide-like) mutagenesis, and survival probability was associated with overall mutation burden and neoantigen load.

Analysis of mRNA expression clustering identified five luminal and basal subtypes, similar to those seen in breast cancer, that stratify outcomes, suggesting different strategies for the use of neoadjuvant chemotherapy, immunotherapy and targeted therapies. Several groups have described similar stratification using expression-based subtyping, as summarized in a recent review.[11]

Molecular profiling is likely to provide useful information about the biology of bladder cancer, including clues to treatment selection and sequencing. For example, responses to atezolizumab are most common in TCGA cluster II cancers; potential driver mutations in *FGFR3* are most common in TCGA cluster I; microsatellite instability, DNA repair defects and altered expression of specific genes such as *APLNR* loss may be important for response to immunotherapy.[12] However, this information has yet to lead to changes in clinical practice.

Patterns of recurrence and spread

Most Ta and T1 tumors can be completely resected cystoscopically and treated successfully without cystectomy. In approximately 40% of patients with such tumors there is no recurrence after resection of the primary tumor; however, this subgroup of patients cannot be initially distinguished with certainty from those whose tumors will recur (stratification criteria are shown in Table 5.2). Among patients who do experience recurrence, 20–30% of tumors (usually high grade) may progress to a higher stage. Thus, vigilant surveillance is necessary, as is judicious use of intravesical agents (see page 45) to decrease the likelihood of recurrence and progression in high-risk patients (e.g. those with large or multiple tumors, high-grade tumors, or Ta or T1 tumors with associated CIS).

Most recurrences occur in the bladder, although 4–10% of patients develop a tumor in the upper urinary tract (ureter and renal pelvis) and a similar number may develop a tumor in the prostatic urethra, which is lined by urothelium similar to that of the bladder. Conversely, 40% of patients who have an initial UC of the renal pelvis will subsequently develop a UC in the bladder.

CIS has a high rate of progression to muscle-invasive disease if it is not eradicated with intravesical therapy, usually bacillus Calmette–Guérin (BCG).

On average, muscle-invasive disease is associated with regional lymph node metastases in 25% of patients. Hematogenous spread is most common to the lungs, liver and bones, and these are the most common sites of progression in patients who experience recurrence after definitive loco-regional therapy with radical cystectomy or chemoradiation. Distant metastases are present at initial diagnosis in 5% of patients.

Mortality

Mortality due to UC is directly related to the pathological stage and grade of bladder cancer (Table 2.2).[13] For those with low-grade Ta and T1 tumors, 5-year disease-specific survival should exceed 95%, whereas reported 5-year survival may be as low as 50% for patients with high-grade T1 cancers or CIS without adjuvant therapy. Intravesical immunotherapy with BCG is associated with frequent complete response at 6 months following induction and initial maintenance, and 5-year survival should approach 80–85%. For patients with T2/T3aN0M0 disease, the 5-year survival rate is 60–70%, despite radical cystectomy. Progression is often due to subclinical 'micrometastases' that were present at the time of cystectomy but were not radiologically detectable. In patients who experience disease progression, this occurs within 2–3 years of cystectomy in about 80% of cases. Patients who are treated with peri-operative chemotherapy may experience late relapse (after 5 years), with metastases often occurring at unusual sites, including the central nervous system or intraperitoneally, presenting as bowel obstruction.

The 5-year survival rate in patients with T4 UC is only 10–20%; survival of those with T4a disease is at the upper end of this range. The 5-year survival rate for individuals with para-aortic or distant lymph node metastases but no visceral disease is 20–40%, although occasionally cure is possible with chemotherapy. For patients with visceral metastases the 5-year survival rate, irrespective of chemotherapy, is only about 10%. Independent adverse prognostic determinants for patients with metastatic disease include poor performance status, weight loss and raised liver function test results and alkaline phosphatase levels. Sex and age are not independent prognostic variables.

Patients with adenocarcinoma or squamous carcinoma have a 5-year survival rate of more than 50% following radical cystectomy, provided that the lymph nodes are negative. Urachal adenocarcinoma is treated with partial cystectomy, and adjuvant therapy for locally advanced cancers is similar to the treatment for colon cancer. However, if metastases are present, the prognosis is grim (see page 62). Patients with small-cell neuroendocrine carcinoma may be cured with systemic chemotherapy and cystectomy or radiation if there is no residual small-cell carcinoma. The prognosis for bladder sarcomas is determined by histological subtype, extent of disease and performance status.

TABLE 2.2

Five-year survival rates for patients with various stages of urothelial carcinoma

Grade	Five-year survival rate
Low-grade Ta or T1	>95%
High-grade T1 or CIS	
Without treatment	50%
With treatment	80–85%
T2/T3aN0M0	60–70%
T4	10–20%
Para-aortic or distant lymph node metastases	
Without visceral disease	20–40%
With visceral disease	10%

CIS, Carcinoma in situ

Key points – pathology and biology

- Urothelial carcinoma is the predominant histology of bladder cancer.
- Variant histology is common and is usually seen as a mixed pattern with conventional urothelial cancer.
- Low-grade non-muscle-invasive bladder tumors may recur but progression to muscle invasion occurs in <5% of cases.
- High-grade non-muscle-invasive bladder cancer will progress if not adequately treated with resection and intravesical therapy.
- Carcinoma in situ, whether primary or associated with Ta or T1 papillary tumor, is a high-risk cancer.
- Up to 30% of patients with high-grade non-muscle-invasive tumors and up to 70% with muscle-invasive disease may die of bladder cancer.

Key references

1. Lerner SP, Schoenberg M, Sternberg C, eds. *Treatment and Management of Bladder Cancer*. London: Wiley-Blackwell, 2015.

2. Khaled H. Schistosomiasis and cancer in Egypt: review. *J Adv Res* 2013;4:461–6.

3. Shokeir AA. Squamous cell carcinoma of the bladder: pathology, diagnosis and treatment. *BJU Int* 2004;93:216–20.

4. Siefker-Radtke AO, Gee J, Shen Y et al. Multimodality management of urachal carcinoma: the M. D. Anderson Cancer Center experience. *J Urol* 2003;169:1295–8.

5. Ching CB, Amin MB, Tubbs RR et al. HER2 gene amplification occurs frequently in the micropapillary variant of urothelial carcinoma: analysis by dual-color in situ hybridization. *Mod Pathol* 2011;24:1111–19.

6. Keck B, Stoehr R, Wach S et al. The plasmacytoid carcinoma of the bladder – rare variant of aggressive urothelial carcinoma. *Int J Cancer* 2011;129:346–54.

7. Eble JN, Sauter G, Epstein JI, Sesterhenn IA, eds. *World Health Organization Classification of Tumours: Pathology and Genetics of Tumours of the Urinary and Male Genital Organs*. Lyon: IARC Press, 2004.

8. Amin MB, Edge S, Byrd D et al, eds. *AJCC Cancer Staging Manual*. Heidelberg, Springer, 2017.

9. Knowles MA, Hurst CD. Molecular biology of bladder cancer: new insights into pathogenesis and clinical diversity. *Nat Rev Cancer* 2015;15:25–41.

10. Robertson AG, Kim J, Al-Ahmadie H et al. Comprehensive molecular characterization of muscle-invasive bladder cancer. *Cell* 2017;171:540–56 e25.

11. Kamat AM, Hahn NM, Efstathiou JA et al. Bladder cancer. *Lancet* 2016;388:2796–810.

12. Patel SJ, Sanjana NE, Kishton RJ et al. Identification of essential genes for cancer immunotherapy. *Nature* 2017;548:537–42.

13. Cancer Research UK. *Bladder cancer statistics*. 2017. www.cancerresearchuk.org/health-professional/cancer-statistics/statistics-by-cancer-type/bladder-cancer. Last accessed 30 January 2018.

3 Clinical presentation

The classic presenting sign or symptom of a bladder tumor is painless gross or microscopic hematuria; it is the sole presenting symptom in 60–80% of patients. Unfortunately, and despite the well-known sinister implications of this finding, many patients who present with hematuria are not evaluated further or referred to a urologist.[1,2] Up to 20% of patients with bladder cancer will not have hematuria at presentation. Other patterns of presentation also occur (Table 3.1) and are sometimes similarly unrecognized as an indication of serious underlying pathology.

Computed tomographic urography (CTU) is the imaging modality of choice for the evaluation of hematuria and the detection of urothelial cancer.[3,4] Magnetic resonance urography is an alternative for patients who cannot receive intravenous iodinated contrast.[5,6]

Painless hematuria

Painless hematuria may occur at the beginning, end or throughout the urine stream. It may be profuse (such that the patient describes passing pure blood) and contain clots or it may have only a slight pink discoloration. Clots that have been in the bladder for some time may impart a rusty color to the urine. Any patient with these symptoms should be referred to a urologist immediately.

Urinary tract bleeding is intermittent with spontaneous resolution, so a single episode warrants evaluation. However, patients sometimes ignore a single episode of hematuria and do not seek advice until the bleeding recurs. Menstruating women may also sometimes confuse hematuria with menstrual flow. The resultant delay in diagnosis and treatment may make treatment more difficult and reduce the possibility of cure.

Asymptomatic microscopic hematuria

The finding of microscopic or dipstick hematuria is increasing as screening programs and medical examinations for insurance purposes

TABLE 3.1

Presenting symptoms

Symptom	Description
Painless hematuria	Visible passage of blood in urine, without associated pain, frequency or dysuria
	Particularly significant for men and postmenopausal women
	Up to 10% of patients with painless hematuria will have urinary tract malignancy
Microscopic hematuria	Presence of red blood cells in the urine of insufficient quantity to be visible to the naked eye, without urologic symptoms
	About 4–6% of patients will have urinary tract malignancy
Irritative symptoms	Dysuria, frequency, nocturia, suprapubic pain with a full bladder
	About 25% of patients with bladder tumors have one or more of these symptoms
Recurrent urinary tract infection	The possibility of an underlying tumor should be considered in older patients (≥ 50 years) with recurrent bacterial cystitis
Symptoms of local or distant spread	Loin pain, weight loss, malaise, anorexia, bone pain, pathological fracture, cough, headache, abdominal pain

become more widespread. Significant microscopic hematuria is defined as three or more red blood cells per high-power field on a properly collected urine sample, in the absence of a benign cause.[3] There is good correlation of 1+ or more dipstick hematuria with significant microscopic hematuria. Abnormal dipstick hematuria results should be confirmed by microscopic examination. Microscopic hematuria may be part of the spectrum of painless hematuria; however, the sensitivity and specificity of a single urinalysis is low for detection of bladder cancer.

Irritative symptoms

Irritative symptoms such as dysuria, increased frequency and urgency are often dismissed because they are common, are usually due to urinary tract infection (UTI) and are typically not associated with serious disease. However, if infection is absent or symptoms persist after the UTI has been treated, the possibility of an underlying bladder malignancy must be considered and the patient referred to a urologist.

Irritative symptoms are particularly common in patients with carcinoma in situ (CIS), and suprapubic pain when the bladder is full can also be caused by carcinoma of the bladder.

Urinalysis in patients with irritative symptoms due to CIS or invasive cancer will usually reveal the presence of red or white blood cells. Urine cytology, if it is considered and requested, may detect malignant cells.

Recurrent urinary tract infections

Recurrent UTI is sometimes due to the presence of a bladder tumor. A single UTI in a man, or two or more in a woman, should be investigated; however, the likelihood of a malignant etiology is very low in patients under 50 years of age.

Symptoms of local or distant spread

Patients sometimes present with systemic symptoms due to advanced carcinoma of the bladder. Loin pain can be caused by ureteric obstruction due to an invasive bladder tumor (Figure 3.1). The pain is usually a dull ache in the costophrenic angle, and may or may not coincide with other symptoms such as hematuria. Occasionally, infection occurs in an obstructed system, giving rise to severe symptoms of pyelonephritis.

Coughing, dyspnea or chest pain may be due to pulmonary metastases (Figure 3.2); the cough is usually non-productive. Pleuritic chest pain may also be present.

Anorexia, nausea, weight loss and malaise may result from renal failure due to bilateral ureteric obstruction, or from the systemic effects of the tumor itself. Bone pain or pathological fractures may result from skeletal metastases (Figure 3.3); the pain is unrelieved by rest and can be severe. Anemia and hypercalcemia may occur as

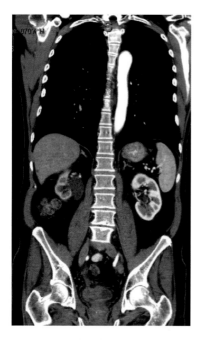

Figure 3.1 Computed tomography urogram showing ureteric obstruction by a bladder tumor. Obstruction is a sign of an invasive tumor.

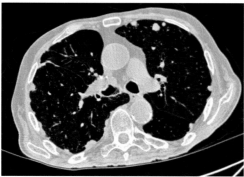

Figure 3.2 Chest computed tomography showing multiple pulmonary metastases.

metabolic complications of advanced disease; leukocytosis is occasionally associated with the elaboration of colony-stimulating factors by the tumor.

Headache or disordered thought processes are uncommon as a presenting feature but may indicate underlying brain metastases or carcinomatous meningitis.

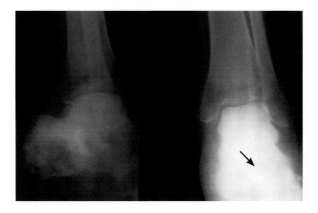

Figure 3.3 Bone destruction by secondary deposits from an invasive bladder tumor. Pathological fracture may occur if deposits occur in a weight-bearing bone.

Delay in diagnosis

Although it is difficult to prove that delay in diagnosis affects prognosis, screening for asymptomatic microscopic hematuria is associated with a shift towards more favorable tumor characteristics of lower stage and grade at diagnosis, and better survival.[7] Delays may occur for a variety of reasons.[8]

- Presentation by the patient may be delayed because of anxiety about the cause of the symptoms, fear of primary care physicians or hospitals or ignorance of the significance of symptoms.
- Referral by the primary care physician to a specialist may be delayed because of ignorance of the significance of the symptoms, or limited access to specialist healthcare (waiting times for clinic appointments).
- Diagnosis by the specialist may be delayed because of waiting times for investigations, follow-up clinic appointments for results, or cystoscopy.

Taken together, these factors mean that the average time from the first symptom to treatment of the bladder tumor varies from a few weeks to more than a year across studies.

In an attempt to streamline the diagnosis and treatment of patients with symptoms suggestive of bladder cancer, many hospitals now offer a hematuria clinic at which patients can be seen within a week of referral. The service should be able to perform urine cytology and dipstick analysis for blood and leukocytes, CTU or renal ultrasonography and plain radiography of the urinary tract, and flexible cystoscopy, all on the same day. This allows a diagnosis to be made and treatment planned expeditiously.

Key points – clinical presentation

- Painless hematuria is the most common presentation of bladder cancer.
- A single episode of hematuria should prompt urgent referral to a urologist.
- Unexplained irritative symptoms may be due to bladder cancer, particularly carcinoma in situ.
- Recurrent infections may indicate an underlying tumor.
- Delay in treatment adversely affects prognosis.
- Hematuria clinics allow rapid diagnosis and reduce time to treatment.

Key references

1. Ark JT, Alvarez JR, Koyama T et al. Variation in the diagnostic evaluation among persons with hematuria: influence of gender, race and risk factors for bladder cancer. *J Urol* 2017;198:1033–8.

2. Elias K, Svatek RS, Gupta S et al. High-risk patients with hematuria are not evaluated according to guideline recommendations. *Cancer* 2010;116:2954–9.

3. Davis R, Jones JS, Barocas DA et al. Diagnosis, evaluation and follow-up of asymptomatic microhematuria (AMH) in adults: AUA guideline. *J Urol* 2012;188:2473–81.

4. Silverman SG, Leyendecker JR, Amis ES, Jr. What is the current role of CT urography and MR urography in the evaluation of the urinary tract? *Radiology* 2009;250:309–23.

5. Leyendecker JR, Barnes CE, Zagoria RJ. MR urography: techniques and clinical applications. *Radiographics* 2008;28:23–46; discussion 46–7.

6. Lee KS, Zeikus E, DeWolf WC et al. MR urography versus retrograde pyelography/ureteroscopy for the exclusion of upper urinary tract malignancy. *Clin Radiol* 2010;65:185–92.

7. Madeb R, Messing EM. Long-term outcome of home dipstick testing for hematuria. *World J Urol* 2008;26:19–24.

8. Hayne D, Stockler M, McCombie SP et al. BCG + Mitomycin trial for high-risk non-muscle-invasive bladder cancer: progress report and lessons learned. *BJU Int* 2017;119(Suppl 5):5–7.

Investigations

History

A thorough history should be obtained from any patient presenting with symptoms suggestive of bladder cancer. The history should cover smoking, occupational history (including possible carcinogen exposure in the workplace), previous bladder tumor resection and any change in bowel habits or stool characteristics. Direct questioning may reveal hematuria for 6–12 months prior to presentation.

Examination

Physical examination is usually unremarkable in cases of non-muscle-invasive bladder cancer (NMIBC) unless acute urinary retention is present with bladder distension. In men, a careful rectal examination should be carried out to exclude prostatic disease such as cancer or benign enlargement, both of which may cause many of the same symptoms as bladder cancer, and to rule out gross extension of bladder cancer into the prostate. A careful pelvic examination in women is equally important. A thorough nodal examination should be undertaken, including the supraclavicular lymph nodes, as well as assessment for hepatic or pulmonary involvement.

Detailed investigation

Urinalysis should begin with dipstick testing for the presence of red blood cells. If the result is positive, microscopic analysis should be performed for confirmation. The presence of nitrates or leukocytes should prompt urine culture to look for infection.

Tests for urinary markers of urothelial malignancy have recently become commercially available, although tests for other urinary markers are still at the laboratory stage.[1]

    Bladder tumor antigen (BTA) stat® test is performed on unmodified (unbuffered) urine using a similar method to pregnancy tests, and results are available within 5 minutes. The second-generation BTA stat test detects a different protein from that detected by the original test, and has better sensitivity but similar specificity. The test, which can be performed at the time of cystoscopy, is claimed to be approximately twice as sensitive as cytology, and is particularly effective for detecting the low- and intermediate-grade tumors that cytology misses.

In the UK, surveillance cystoscopy is usually performed in the outpatient setting using a flexible (diagnostic only) cystoscope. One study showed substantial cost savings if patients with a positive BTA stat test result did not undergo flexible cystoscopy but instead were taken directly to anesthesia and rigid cystoscopy for possible resection, even allowing for a few with negative results on rigid cystoscopy (i.e. false-positive BTA stat tests). Some reports indicate that the BTA stat test may be more useful than cytology; however, this opinion remains controversial. Trials will determine the role of the BTA stat test and whether it can indeed reduce the use of cystoscopy.

BTA TRAK® is a quantitative test that measures the same protein as that detected by the BTA stat test. The level of tumor-associated protein appears to correlate directly with increasing stage and grade of tumor. This test may therefore allow serial follow-up of patients, and indicate response to therapy and prognosis for recurring disease.

NMP22® assay. This test measures a nuclear matrix protein (NMP) secreted by some bladder tumors. NMPs are involved in DNA replication and RNA synthesis and are released during cell death and can be detected in the blood and in urine. NMP22 is present in transitional cell tumors and can be detected by immunoassay. The test has to be performed in a laboratory.

The BTA stat, BTA TRAK, NMP22, BladderChek® and UroVysion® tests are approved by the US Food and Drug Administration for use in the evaluation of hematuria as an adjunct to cystoscopy. They may also be useful in dictating the frequency of cystoscopy for recurrence in patients with known bladder cancer. Table 4.1 shows the sensitivity and specificity of some of these markers. Current consensus is that none of the tests alone is sufficiently sensitive to replace cystoscopy in diagnosing or excluding urinary bladder cancer.

Imaging. The upper tracts (ureter and renal pelvis) should be imaged in all patients with symptoms suggestive of bladder cancer. In the

TABLE 4.1

Sensitivity and specificity of tests for urinary markers of bladder cancer

Test	Sensitivity (%)	Specificity (%)	Comment
Cytology	49.8	96.6	Readily available
BTA stat®	67.7	65.8	False positives with infection/hematuria
BTA TRAK®	71.1	62.0	Complex test*
NMP22®	64.3	71.2	Complex test*
UroVysion®	79	88	Complex test*
Telomerase	74	89	Complex test,* not commercially available
HA/HAase	91	86	Complex test,* not commercially available
Immunocyt™	68	79	Complex test*

*Requires reference laboratory.
BTA, bladder tumor antigen; HA/HAase, hyaluronic acid/hyaluronidase; NMP, nuclear matrix protein.

investigation of hematuria (the most common presentation of bladder cancer), contemporary imaging can be performed by computed tomographic urography (CTU) (Figure 4.1),[2,3] which has replaced intravenous urography. Renal ultrasonography plus a plain radiograph of the kidneys, ureters and bladder is an option when CTU is not available and if the patient cannot receive intravenous contrast. Retrograde ureteropyelography should be used to resolve any abnormalities on non-contrast studies. Magnetic resonance urography is another option, particularly for patients with an allergy to iodinated intravenous contrast and for pregnant women.[4] It has 69% sensitivity and 97% specificity for upper-tract tumors. As radiological imaging cannot sufficiently evaluate the bladder, cystoscopy is a required part of the evaluation for all patients.

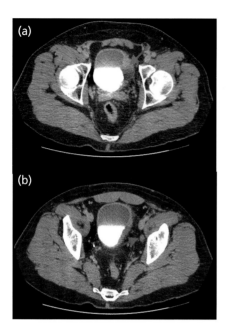

Figure 4.1 Computed tomography urograms showing (a) high grade invasive cancer left lateral wall, (b) left internal iliac lymph node metastasis.

If a patient is found to have low-grade bladder cancer on biopsy, no further imaging is required. High-risk NMIBC can be associated with occult lymph node metastases, and computed tomography (CT) or magnetic resonance imaging (MRI) may be considered in these patients. However, if muscle-invasive disease is present, staging with chest, abdominal and pelvic CT is necessary. This should identify any visceral metastatic disease within the limits of resolution of the scanner. Pelvic MRI scanning may give more accurate information about the local spread of an invasive tumor.

Bone scans are indicated only for patients with invasive disease who have symptoms suggesting bone involvement (i.e. pain) or in the presence of elevated bone markers (alkaline phosphatase).

Cystoscopy is required in all patients in order to evaluate the bladder. It can usually be accomplished in the ambulatory urology clinic without anesthesia, using a flexible cystoscope. Diagnostic cystoscopy may be omitted if a bladder tumor is obvious on cross-sectional imaging; however, most urologists perform the procedure in order to inform surgical management, and it allows the patient to be informed of the likely diagnosis of bladder cancer.

When a bladder tumor is identified by imaging or cystoscopy, the next step is to perform a transurethral resection of bladder tumor (TURBT) under general anesthesia using a rigid cystoscope. All visible papillary disease should be completely resected in the case of a probable NMIBC. Site-directed biopsy of remote normal-appearing mucosa is indicated only for high-grade tumors.[5] In patients with an apparent muscle invasive bladder cancer (MIBC), the goals are to establish the histological subtype and depth of penetration and to exclude involvement of the urethra. A pelvic examination under general anesthesia prior to resection aids determination of the clinical stage. Maximal resection is desired if radiation-based treatment is being considered for a patient with MIBC.[6]

Cytological examination of exfoliated cells is part of the hematuria evaluation for all patients. When a bladder tumor is diagnosed, cytology is useful to determine the grade as, by definition, positive cytology denotes high-grade malignant cells. A bladder wash for cytology should be obtained at the time of cystoscopy, as this is the most sensitive means for detection of bladder cancer particularly if areas that might be carcinoma in situ (CIS) or ulcers rather than obvious papillary or exophytic solid tumor are seen. Cytology may be helpful in following up such patients for signs of recurrence, as well as for ensuring that all disease present at initial diagnosis has been diagnosed and treated adequately.

Cytology is relatively insensitive in low-grade disease. Note that cytological evaluation of urine may be compromised if performed soon after urinary tract instrumentation.

Expert pathological interpretation of both histology and cytology specimens is critical. Recent reports indicate a rate of discordance of at least 30% among pathologists, including many who specialize in uropathology. Because many treatment and prognostic decisions are based on fine distinctions between grade (3 versus 1 or 2), depth of invasion (T1 versus T2) and field changes (CIS versus mild or moderate dysplasia), it is important that both understaging and overstaging of bladder cancers is minimized. Second-opinion pathology should be routine if the initial reporting pathologist sees only an occasional case of bladder cancer.

Transurethral resection of the tumor(s) is the mainstay of both diagnosis and initial management. If papillary disease is limited, as is usually the case, additional therapy may not be required, other than regular cystoscopic surveillance (see page 48). The use of peri-operative single-dose intravesical chemotherapy is discussed on page 45. Complete resection may be possible if the tumor is small, papillary or solid, and even if it has invaded the muscle (Figure 4.2). However, extensive resections of large invasive tumors may serve no useful purpose, because cystectomy may be needed shortly. In addition, the risk of postoperative bleeding and clot retention is increased. Deep biopsy at the juncture of the tumor and the muscular wall may be sufficient to confirm the diagnosis of muscle involvement.

Biopsy. Mucosal biopsies should be performed in selected cases to rule out or diagnose associated field changes (see page 19) in the case of high-grade cancers (Figure 4.3). Small, obviously low-grade papillary and superficial tumors do not warrant such biopsies, however.

Biopsy should be performed under the following circumstances:

- multiple papillary tumors
- tumors that appear solid but are resectable
- bladders with erythematous areas that may represent CIS
- if chemoradiation with bladder conservation is being considered
- to determine whether the prostate/bladder neck is free of CIS in patients for whom orthotopic bladder reconstruction is planned after cystectomy.

Biopsies might also be obtained circumferentially around small, solid, apparently invasive tumors away from the bladder base or bladder neck in selected cases where partial cystectomy might be considered for definitive therapy.

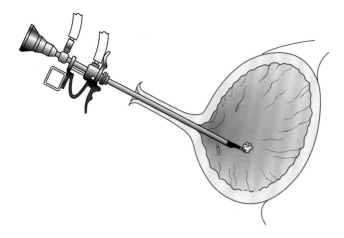

Figure 4.2 Transurethral resection of a small, solid, muscle-invasive tumor.

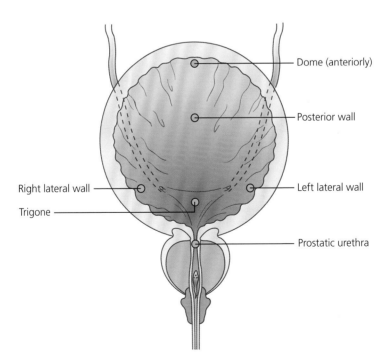

Figure 4.3 Sites for directed mucosal biopsies of the bladder.

Key points – investigations

- The investigation of a patient with suspected bladder cancer should include urinalysis, cross-sectional upper-tract imaging and cystoscopy.
- Expert pathological review of biopsy specimens is critical to determining appropriate treatment.
- Cross-sectional imaging (computed tomography or magnetic resonance imaging) is used to stage invasive disease.
- Urinary markers are not yet sufficiently sensitive for diagnosis but may be useful in following up patients with superficial disease.

Key references

1. Herman MP, Svatek RS, Lotan Y et al. Urine-based biomarkers for the early detection and surveillance of non-muscle invasive bladder cancer. *Minerva Urol Nefrol* 2008;60:217–35.

2. Silverman SG, Leyendecker JR, Amis ES, Jr. What is the current role of CT urography and MR urography in the evaluation of the urinary tract? *Radiology* 2009;250:309–23.

3. Davis R, Jones JS, Barocas DA et al. Diagnosis, evaluation and follow-up of asymptomatic microhematuria (AMH) in adults: AUA guideline. *J Urol* 2012;188:2473–81.

4. Leyendecker JR, Barnes CE, Zagoria RJ. MR urography: techniques and clinical applications. *Radiographics* 2008;28:23–46; discussion 46–7.

5. Power NE, Izawa J. Comparison of guidelines on non-muscle invasive bladder cancer (EAU, CUA, AUA, NCCN, NICE). *Bladder Cancer* 2016;2:27–36.

6. Chang SS, Bochner BH, Chou R et al. Treatment of non-metastatic muscle-invasive bladder cancer: AUA/ASCO/ASTRO/SUO guideline. *J Urol* 2017;198:552–9.

Basic principles

The majority of patients (70%) initially present with non-muscle invasive bladder cancer (NMIBC). Treatment is based on a risk-stratified approach that takes into account multiple prognostic factors associated with a risk of recurrence and progression to muscle-invasive disease. Intravesical chemotherapy with mitomycin and immunotherapy with bacillus Calmette–Guérin (BCG) are the most commonly used approaches. Treatment of NMIBC involves the multi-step interventional strategies summarized in Table 5.1.

Initial surgical management

Pathological diagnosis is established by transurethral resection of bladder tumor (TURBT) and biopsy of abnormal-appearing adjacent or remote bladder mucosa. The goal of this endoscopic surgery is to

TABLE 5.1

Multi-step interventional strategies used in the treatment of non-muscle-invasive bladder cancer

Stage	Role of intravesical treatment
Macroablation (TURBT)	Intravesical chemotherapy or immunotherapy have limited roles because all visible papillary disease should be resected prior to therapy
Re-implantation post-TURBT	Peri-operative single-dose intravesical chemotherapy
Microablation for subclinical residual disease (e.g. carcinoma in situ)	Chemo/immunotherapy has a major role

TURBT, transurethral resection of bladder tumor.

41

establish the histology, grade and depth of invasion of the tumor and the presence or absence of carcinoma in situ (CIS), which is often not detectable by white light.

The standard of care for patients with T1 high-grade (HG) disease, uniformly supported by all the guidelines, is repeat resection, in order to determine the completeness of the resection and to rule out a more deeply invasive cancer prior to determination of treatment.[1] Enhanced cystoscopic imaging with fluorescence cystoscopy using pre-operative instillation of 5-aminolevulinic acid or hexylaminolevulinate (Cysview®) improves the detection of papillary and CIS lesions and modestly reduces the recurrence rate.[2,3] Narrow-band imaging is an alternative technique that does not require an imaging agent as it detects hypervascularity associated with bladder tumors. Initial reports suggested a similar association with reduction in recurrence risk[4] but this was not confirmed by a large international trial, except in patients with low-risk disease.[5]

Prognostic factors

Following initial surgical management and determination of stage and grade, the following additional risk factors are assessed:

- tumor size (< 3 cm vs ≥ 3 cm)
- whether this is the first occurrence or a recurrent tumor
- tumor focality (unifocal vs multifocal)
- presence or absence of CIS.

These prognostic factors individually and collectively affect the probability of recurrence and progression and are used to stratify patients into prognostic groups that drive decisions about appropriate treatment and follow-up.

Prognostic groups

Patients are stratified into risk groups for progression, based on low grade to high grade or non-invasive to invasive cancer. Most risk stratification schemes use three strata: low, intermediate and high risk, as illustrated by the American Urological Association system presented in Table 5.2.[6] The European Association of Urology adds a highest-risk group which should be treated with radical cystectomy. This group includes HG T1 associated with concurrent CIS, multiple and/or large HG T1 and/or recurrent HG T1, HG T1 with CIS in the prostatic urethra, unusual histology of urothelial carcinoma and lympho-vascular invasion.[7]

The risk strata inform decisions about the use of adjuvant therapy and surveillance schedules. Power and Izawa have compared and contrasted current NMIBC guideline recommendations.[1] A calculator based on European Organisation for Research and Treatment of Cancer clinical trials (eortc.be/tools/bladdercalculator) is a useful tool for risk stratification.[8]

Low-risk tumors. Patients with a solitary low-grade Ta lesion are at low risk of recurrence or progression. Level-I evidence supports use of peri-operative single-dose chemotherapy, with an 11% absolute reduction in recurrence and a 39% relative risk reduction.[9] Mitomycin is the most commonly used drug in this setting, and epirubicin is available in Europe.[10] The recent report of the SWOG S-0337 trial provides additional level-I evidence for the use of gemcitabine.[11] Induction chemotherapy (intravesical therapy weekly for 6 weeks) is not indicated for patients with low-risk disease. Furthermore, recent

TABLE 5.2

American Urological Association risk stratification for bladder cancer (2016)[6]

Low risk	Intermediate risk	High risk
LG solitary Ta ≤ 3 cm	Recurrence within 1 year, LG Ta	HG T1
Papillary urothelial neoplasm of low malignant potential	Solitary LG Ta > 3 cm	Any recurrent HG Ta
	LG Ta, multifocal	HG Ta > 3cm (or multifocal)
	HG Ta, ≤ 3 cm	Any carcinoma in situ
	LG T1	Any BCG failure in HG
		Any variant histology
		Any lymphovascular invasion
		Any HG prostatic urethral involvement

BCG, bacillus Calmette–Guérin; HG, high grade; LG, low grade.

experience suggests that if the first surveillance cystoscopy is negative, the interval to the next cystoscopy can be extended to 9 months (rather than 3 months), with annual cystoscopy thereafter.

Patients who develop a recurrence of similar stage and grade are classified as intermediate risk and have been shown to benefit from intravesical chemotherapy.

Intermediate-risk tumors. Patients with multiple or recurrent low-grade Ta tumors are at intermediate risk of recurrence or progression. Small-volume Ta HG cancers are included in this risk stratum in the American Urological Association scheme (Table 5.2). Patients with frequent recurrences of low-grade Ta tumors require cystoscopic resection for each recurrence: this interferes with the patient's life; however, this stage does not usually threaten life or bladder preservation. These patients should receive a course of intravesical therapy following resection (see below). Mitomycin is the most commonly used cytotoxic drug. BCG induction plus maintenance for 1 year is also an option.[12]

High-risk tumors. Patients who present with CIS and/or HG papillary tumors (Ta or T1) have an 80% risk of recurrence and progression rates of 40–70%. BCG is the standard of care; level-I evidence supports induction therapy weekly for 6 weeks, followed by maintenance treatment weekly for 3 weeks at months 3 and 6 and then at 6-month intervals to 3 years.[12,13] Disease that recurs or persists after one course of BCG has a greater likelihood of progressing; however, approximately one-third of such patients respond to a second induction course. Recurrence with a HG tumor after two induction courses (6 weeks + 6 weeks) or induction plus first maintenance therapy (6 weeks + 3 weeks) are deemed BCG unresponsive and should not receive further BCG.[14] Radical cystectomy is the standard of care, supported by multiple guidelines. The US Food and Drug Administration (FDA) has defined a registration pathway based on a single-arm trial that has led to multiple ongoing clinical trials in this disease stage.[15] Valrubicin is currently the only FDA-approved drug for the treatment of BCG-unresponsive CIS in patients who refuse or are deemed medically unfit for cystectomy.[16]

Intravesical therapy

Intravesical administration of chemotherapy and immunotherapeutic agents, delivered into the bladder via a urethral catheter (Figure 5.1), is the primary treatment modality for reducing the risk of recurrence and progression and eradicating CIS. Commonly used agents with demonstrated activity include thiotepa, docetaxel, doxorubicin, epirubicin, gemcitabine, interferon, mitomycin and valrubicin. Historically, doxorubicin and mitomycin have been the preferred agents because systemic absorption is limited by their high molecular mass. Thiotepa has a low molecular mass, increasing the risk of absorption through a denuded urothelium, with a potential risk of bone marrow suppression. Optimal treatment requires complete resection of all visible papillary disease (Ta and T1) before initiating intravesical therapy. BCG provides optimal therapeutic benefit for the eradication of CIS.

Chemotherapy. Optimal delivery of mitomycin is achieved by doubling the dose and concentration compared with historical doses of 20 mg/20 mL sterile water. An 'optimized' treatment algorithm supported by level-I evidence includes the following additional measures:[17]

- alkalinizing the urine by the oral administration of bicarbonate on the evening before and the morning of treatment
- minimizing the residual urine after catheterization of the bladder
- keeping the patient fasted throughout treatment in order to minimize urine production.

These measures effectively doubled the 5-year recurrence-free survival, from 25% to 50%. The absorption of mitomycin may be optimized by the delivery of heat or iontophoresis.[18,19] Monthly maintenance treatment for 10 months reduces the probability of recurrence in patients who have an initial complete response.[20]

Single-agent gemcitabine and docetaxel have demonstrated efficacy in disease that is refractory to initial treatment with other agents, and the two drugs have been used in combination effectively in patients with BCG-unresponsive disease, particularly CIS.[21,22]

Intravesical immunotherapy with BCG was first reported to decrease papillary tumor recurrence in 1976.[23] BCG is an attenuated strain of

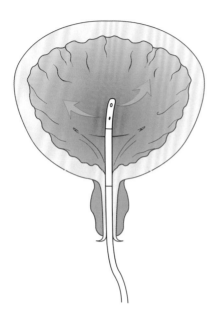

Figure 5.1 Intravesical therapy. The agent is instilled into the bladder via a disposable catheter and must be retained within the bladder for 2 hours. The patient may be asked to change position frequently from lying on one side to the other and supine to prone, in order to coat the bladder and then to remain ambulatory for the remainder of the time, followed by spontaneous voiding to eliminate the agent. This changing of position and prolonged retention is important because bacillus Calmette–Guérin works by attaching to the bladder mucosa, and absorption of most chemotherapy agents is driven by a concentration gradient.

Mycobacterium bovis that stimulates an immune response without causing tuberculosis. The bacillus acts as a non-specific promoter of cellular immunity in the urothelium, activating cytotoxic lymphocytes and stimulating release of various tumoricidal cytokines, working in part through the induction of interferon gamma. BCG is the most effective agent for prevention of both recurrence and tumor progression. BCG immunotherapy is also highly effective in CIS: induction plus maintenance therapy results in complete remission of disease in up to 85% of patients.[13]

A disadvantage of BCG is its toxicity, which is greater than that of intravesical chemotherapy (Table 5.3) and may be substantial during maintenance courses. For this reason, BCG immunotherapy is generally used only for first-line treatment in patients with high-risk disease, and as a second-line therapy for patients with intermediate-risk disease that continues to recur after adequate intravesical chemotherapy. Some of the side effects of BCG may be prevented or decreased in severity, without affecting effectiveness, through the concomitant administration of quinolones with each intravesical treatment.[24,25] BCG is contraindicated in the presence of gross hematuria, traumatic catheterization or immune suppression, as these increase the risk of potentially life-threatening intravascular dissemination.

Given the success of BCG immunotherapy, several other immunotherapeutic agents have been investigated. The most clinical experience has been gathered for recombinant interferon alfa-2b (Intron A®, Schering Plough) and bropirimine. Glashan first reported a complete response in 45% of patients with CIS following intravesical administration of interferon alfa-2b, 100 mega units weekly for 12 weeks.[27]

While BCG alone is the standard of care for patients with a first occurrence of a high-risk tumor,[28] BCG in combination with interferon may be useful for patients with disease recurrence after an initial course of BCG.[29]

TABLE 5.3

Complications of intravesical therapy*

Complication	BCG (n = 2062)[26]	Chemotherapy
Fever	2.9 (75)[†]	0
Granulomatous prostatitis	0.9 (23)	0
Pneumonitis/hepatitis	0.7 (18)	(3)[‡]
Arthralgia	0.5 (12)	0
Hematuria	0.9 (24)	Rare
Rash	0.3 (8)	9
Ureteral obstruction	0.3 (8)	(4)[‡]
Epididymitis	0.4 (10)	0
Contracted bladder	0.2 (6)	0.1
Renal abscess	0.1 (2)	0
Sepsis	0.4 (10)	0
Cytopenia	0.1 (2)	(2)[‡]

*Between 60% and 80% of patients receiving BCG (Bacillus Calmette–Guérin) immunotherapy experience symptoms of cystitis and/or a mild influenza-like illness after each instillation. About 15% of patients report symptoms of cystitis with mitomycin, but it is rarely necessary to stop treatment.
†Values are % (number) of patients; ‡Case reports.

Bropirimine has also been shown to clear CIS in some patients following failure of BCG immunotherapy but it is no longer used as it is not approved by the US FDA because of uncertainties regarding its true anticancer efficacy and concerns about cardiotoxicity.

Surveillance following initial diagnosis and treatment

Cystoscopy. Routine surveillance for NMIBC with cystoscopy can be risk adjusted.
- Patients with a normal cystoscopy 3 months after TURBT for low-risk disease should have a repeat cystoscopy within 9 months and then, if normal, annually thereafter for up to 5 years.
- Intermediate-risk patients should have cystoscopy every 3 months for 1–2 years, then annually for up to 5 years. If recurrence is detected, the patient returns to the start of this schedule.
- Patients with high-risk disease should have cystoscopy every 3 months for 2 years, then every 6 months for a year and annually for up to 5 years thereafter.

As late recurrence can occur, lifelong surveillance is recommended, particularly for patients with high-risk tumors. In the UK, patients who have had low- and intermediate-risk tumors are often discharged from follow-up after 10 years without recurrence. However, they must be told that any future episode of hematuria requires investigation. Lifelong surveillance is usual in the USA but an optimal schedule has not been defined.

Cytology. For patients with HG tumors, either papillary or CIS, voided or bladder wash cytology should be performed as an adjunct to cystoscopy. For low- or intermediate-grade tumors (grade 1 or 2), the yield for cytology is low and routine use is not recommended.

The test is usually performed at the time of cystoscopy, often with a saline wash of the bladder, which has higher sensitivity than with a voided specimen. Results are not available for several days, and some expertise is required to perform the test and interpret the results.

Tumor markers. Various urinary markers for bladder cancer are being evaluated; these are compared in Table 4.1. As yet, no single urinary test has sufficient sensitivity to exclude bladder cancer, so no test can replace cystoscopy in the investigation of a patient with a suspected tumor. However, such tests may reduce the frequency of cystoscopy or inform the appropriate frequency of cystoscopy for recurrence in patients with known bladder cancer.

Key points – management of non-muscle-invasive bladder cancer

- Risk-adapted treatment is based on accurate determination of stage, grade, number of tumors and presence of carcinoma in situ, and stratified as primary versus recurrent disease.
- Tumors can be classified into low-, intermediate- and high-risk based on these factors; these risk strata drive treatment decisions and surveillance recommendations.
- Low-risk tumors may recur but are unlikely to progress. Perioperative single-dose chemotherapy reduces recurrence, and patients may only need cystoscopic follow-up.
- Intermediate-risk tumors are more likely to recur and have a modest progression risk. A course of intravesical chemotherapy will reduce the risk of recurrence but not of progression. Optimized mitomycin treatment is associated with optimal outcomes. Induction with bacillus Calmette–Guérin (BCG) followed by maintenance for 1 year is also a standard of care.
- High-risk bladder cancer is likely to recur and, unless adequately treated, to progress. It is fatal in up to 30% of patients. Intravesical BCG induction plus maintenance for 3 years is standard of care.
- Radical cystectomy is indicated for patients with high-risk disease that is unresponsive to BCG, if the patient is medically fit and accepts the risks.

Key references

1. Power NE, Izawa J. Comparison of guidelines on non-muscle invasive bladder cancer (EAU, CUA, AUA, NCCN, NICE). *Bladder Cancer* 2016;2:27–36.

2. Grossman HB, Stenzl A, Fradet Y et al. Long-term decrease in bladder cancer recurrence with hexaminolevulinate enabled fluorescence cystoscopy. *J Urol* 2012;188:58–62.

3. Stenzl A, Penkoff H, Dajc-Sommerer E et al. Detection and clinical outcome of urinary bladder cancer with 5-aminolevulinic acid-induced fluorescence cystoscopy: a multicenter randomized, double-blind, placebo-controlled trial. *Cancer* 2011;117:938–47.

4. Herr HW, Donat SM. Reduced bladder tumour recurrence rate associated with narrow-band imaging surveillance cystoscopy. *BJU Int* 2011;107:396–8.

5. Naito S, Algaba F, Babjuk M et al. The Clinical Research Office of the Endourological Society (CROES) multicentre randomised trial of narrow band imaging-assisted transurethral resection of bladder tumour (TURBT) versus conventional white light imaging-assisted TURBT in primary non-muscle-invasive bladder cancer patients: trial protocol and 1-year results. *Eur Urol* 2016;70:506–15.

6. Chang SS, Boorjian SA, Chou R et al. Diagnosis and treatment of non-muscle invasive bladder cancer: AUA/SUO guideline. *J Urol* 2016;196:1021–9.

7. Babjuk M, Bohle A, Burger M et al. EAU guidelines on non-muscle-invasive urothelial carcinoma of the bladder: Update 2016. *Eur Urol* 2017;71:447–61.

8. Sylvester RJ, van der Meijden AP, Oosterlinck W et al. Predicting recurrence and progression in individual patients with stage Ta T1 bladder cancer using EORTC risk tables: a combined analysis of 2596 patients from seven EORTC trials. *Eur Urol* 2006;49:466–75; discussion 475–7.

9. Sylvester RJ, Oosterlinck W, van der Meijden AP. A single immediate postoperative instillation of chemotherapy decreases the risk of recurrence in patients with stage Ta T1 bladder cancer: a meta-analysis of published results of randomized clinical trials. *J Urol* 2004;171:2186–90, quiz 2435.

10. Gudjonsson S, Adell L, Merdasa F et al. Should all patients with non-muscle-invasive bladder cancer receive early intravesical chemotherapy after transurethral resection? The results of a prospective randomised multicentre study. *Eur Urol* 2009;55:773–80.

11. Messing E, Tangen C, Lerner S et al. A phase III blinded study of immediate post-TURBT instillation of gemcitabine versus saline in patients with newly diagnosed or occasionally recurring grade I/II non-muscle invasive bladder cancer. *J Urol* 2017;197:e914.

12. Oddens J, Brausi M, Sylvester R et al. Final results of an EORTC-GU cancers group randomized study of maintenance bacillus Calmette-Guérin in intermediate- and high-risk Ta, T1 papillary carcinoma of the urinary bladder: one-third dose versus full dose and 1 year versus 3 years of maintenance. *Eur Urol* 2013;63:462–72.

13. Lamm DL, Blumenstein BA, Crissman JD et al. Maintenance bacillus Calmette-Guerin immunotherapy for recurrent TA, T1 and carcinoma in situ transitional cell carcinoma of the bladder: a randomized Southwest Oncology Group Study. *J Urol* 2000;163:1124–9.

14. Lerner SP, Dinney C, Kamat A et al. Clarification of bladder cancer disease states following treatment of patients with intravesical BCG. *Bladder Cancer* 2015;1:29–30.

15. Jarow J, Maher VE, Tang S et al. Development of systemic and topical drugs to treat non-muscle invasive bladder cancer. *Bladder Cancer* 2015;1:133–6.

16. Dinney CP, Greenberg RE, Steinberg GD. Intravesical valrubicin in patients with bladder carcinoma in situ and contraindication to or failure after bacillus Calmette-Guérin. *Urol Oncol* 2013;31:1635–42.

17. Au JL, Badalament RA, Wientjes MG et al. Methods to improve efficacy of intravesical mitomycin C: results of a randomized phase III trial. *J Natl Cancer Inst* 2001;93:597–604.

18. Di Stasi SM, Giannantoni A, Stephen RL et al. Intravesical electromotive mitomycin C versus passive transport mitomycin C for high risk superficial bladder cancer: a prospective randomized study. *J Urol* 2003;170:777–82.

19. Halachmi S, Moskovitz B, Maffezzini M et al. Intravesical mitomycin C combined with hyperthermia for patients with T1G3 transitional cell carcinoma of the bladder. *Urol Oncol* 2011;29:259–64.

20. Friedrich MG, Pichlmeier U, Schwaibold H et al. Long-term intravesical adjuvant chemotherapy further reduces recurrence rate compared with short-term intravesical chemotherapy and short-term therapy with bacillus Calmette-Guérin (BCG) in patients with non-muscle-invasive bladder carcinoma. *Eur Urol* 2007;52:1123–9.

21. Milbar N, Kates M, Chappidi MR et al. Oncological outcomes of sequential intravesical gemcitabine and docetaxel in patients with non-muscle invasive bladder cancer. *Bladder Cancer* 2017;3:293–303.

22. Velaer KN, Steinberg RL, Thomas LJ et al. Experience with sequential intravesical gemcitabine and docetaxel as salvage therapy for non-muscle invasive bladder cancer. *Curr Urol Rep* 2016;17:38.

23. Morales A, Eidinger D, Bruce AW. Intracavitary bacillus Calmette-Guerin in the treatment of superficial bladder tumors. *J Urol* 1976;116:180–3.

24. Colombel M, Saint F, Chopin D et al. The effect of ofloxacin on bacillus Calmette-Guerin induced toxicity in patients with superficial bladder cancer: results of a randomized, prospective, double-blind, placebo controlled, multicenter study. *J Urol* 2006;176:935–9.

25. Damiano R, De Sio M, Quarto G et al. Short-term administration of prulifloxacin in patients with nonmuscle-invasive bladder cancer: an effective option for the prevention of bacillus Calmette-Guérin-induced toxicity? *BJU Int* 2009;104:633–9.

26. Lamm DL. Complications of bacillus Calmette-Guérin immunotherapy. *Urol Clin North Am* 1992;19:565–72.

27. Glashan RW. A randomized controlled study of intravesical alpha-2b-interferon in carcinoma in situ of the bladder. *J Urol* 1990;144:658–61.

28. Nepple KG, Lightfoot AJ, Rosevear HM et al. Bacillus Calmette-Guérin with or without interferon alpha-2b and megadose versus recommended daily allowance vitamins during induction and maintenance intravesical treatment of nonmuscle invasive bladder cancer. *J Urol* 184:1915–19.

29. Joudi FN, Smith BJ, O'Donnell MA, National BCG-Interferon Phase 2 Investigator Group. Final results from a national multicenter phase II trial of combination bacillus Calmette-Guérin plus interferon alpha-2B for reducing recurrence of superficial bladder cancer. *Urol Oncol* 2006;24:344–8.

6 Management of muscle-invasive disease

Radical cystectomy and pelvic lymphadenectomy

Radical cystectomy and bilateral pelvic lymphadenectomy is indicated for the treatment of:[1]

- T2–T4a cancers
- non-muscle-invasive bladder cancer in the highest risk strata (see page 44)
- disease that is unresponsive to treatment with bacillus Calmette–Guérin (BCG).

The surgery is associated with a very low rate of local pelvic recurrence in patients without lymph node metastasis. Loco-regional and occult distant metastases may be controlled with neoadjuvant or adjuvant chemotherapy (see page 55).

A meticulous bilateral pelvic lymph node dissection that includes the external and internal iliac, obturator and hypogastric lymph nodes should be performed as part of radical or partial cystectomy. Removal of these lymph nodes is crucial for accurate staging and provides potentially curative treatment in patients with N1 or N2 disease.[2,3] Further extended pelvic lymph node dissection, including the presacral, common iliac, paracaval and para-aortic lymph nodes up to or above the aortic bifurcation may provide additional survival benefit.[4,5]

Urethrectomy. Indications for urethrectomy include diffuse carcinoma in situ (CIS), papillary tumor involving the prostatic urethra, prostatic stromal invasion (T4a), and positive apical margin with CIS or frank tumor involvement. Urethral preservation should be considered in women who desire orthotopic neobladder reconstruction, provided that the bladder neck and urethra are not involved. However, a posterior-based T3 tumor or anterior vaginal wall involvement (T4a) are contraindications, as these restrict the ability to obtain an adequate surgical margin. Second primary tumors of the retained urethra may be late events so long-term monitoring is required.

Peri-operative morbidity and mortality remains high with radical cystectomy, even with experienced surgeons operating in high-volume surgical centers. Almost two-thirds of patients will experience at least one complication following radical cystectomy, and up to one-quarter will require re-admission after discharge.[6] Morbidity may significantly limit use of adjuvant chemotherapy following surgery.

In an effort to improve peri-operative outcomes, performance and nutritional status should be optimized before surgery. The principles of the Enhanced Recovery After Surgery (ERAS) protocol, developed from similar protocols in colorectal surgery, include minimizing narcotic use, avoiding large intravenous fluid shifts, early introduction of oral nutrition following surgery, and avoiding cleansing bowel preparation and nasogastric tubes.[7,8] ERAS protocols have demonstrated benefits in the post-operative management of patients undergoing radical cystectomy, with quicker return of bowel function and shorter length of hospital stay.[9] In a randomized Phase IV study in patients undergoing radical cystectomy, alvimopan, a peripheral μ-opioid antagonist, reduced time to resolution of ileus by 1.3 days and length of hospital stay by 2.7 days.[10]

Long-term tumor control outcomes following radical cystectomy vary considerably; 5-year recurrence-free survival rates of 58–62% are reported in contemporary series.[11] Women tend to be diagnosed at later stages of the disease than are men, with a 30–50% higher risk of death.[12] Other risk factors can also affect outcomes in addition to the tumor–node–metastases (TNM) stage, including age, presence of CIS or lymphovascular invasion, and use of peri-operative chemotherapy, and there is considerable variation in outcomes within TNM stages. Nomograms have been developed in an effort to more accurately predict recurrence, cancer-specific survival and overall survival following radical cystectomy.[13,14]

Minimally invasive surgery. Although open radical cystectomy is considered to be the gold standard for treatment of muscle-invasive bladder cancer, recent series have demonstrated the safety of a minimally invasive surgical approach using robotic-assisted radical cystectomy.[15] The aim of this approach is to reduce blood loss, length of hospital stay, and morbidity compared with open surgery, while maintaining long-term tumor control.[16]

Peri-operative treatment for intermediate- or high-risk bladder cancer

Additional treatment approaches should be considered for the management of organ-confined cancer that is at high risk of local or distant recurrence. Adjuvant and neoadjuvant therapy are collectively referred to as perioperative systemic therapies.

Adjuvant therapy refers to additional treatment given after definitive primary treatment, with the intention of destroying microscopic residual cancer cells in order to reduce the risk of local or distant relapse. Most patients who receive adjuvant therapy will not benefit from it: either the cancer has already been cured by primary therapy or micrometastatic disease exists that is already resistant to the planned adjuvant therapy. However, adjuvant therapy is curative in a subgroup of patients. Until these patients can be identified reliably, all eligible patients are treated and may experience the resultant side effects of treatment, even though only a minority will benefit.

Neoadjuvant therapy refers to the use of systemic therapy before definitive primary treatment, in an attempt to downstage the primary tumor, eliminate micrometastatic disease or enhance the efficacy of the primary treatment.

A large number of clinical trials have explored the benefits of perioperative therapies in muscle-invasive bladder cancer. Most data are based on older but well-established chemotherapy regimens used for metastatic disease. Toxicities are generally similar to those seen in the metastatic setting; however, patients who have had incomplete resolution of the adverse effects of surgery are less able to tolerate post-operative chemotherapy. Most individual trials have failed to show a benefit because of issues of study design or, more commonly, lack of statistical power or slow and incomplete accrual. Systematic reviews, pooled analyses and meta-analyses have been required to demonstrate the purported benefits. This complex literature is summarized in Table 6.1.[17–20]

TABLE 6.1

Summary of the literature relating to adjuvant and neoadjuvant chemotherapy

Adjuvant chemotherapy	• Aligns with conventional clinical management workflow (surgery as the first approach) but might not be the optimal approach
	• Requires a functional multidisciplinary team
	• Overall hazard ratio for survival 0.75 (95% CI 0.60–0.96), $p = 0.019$)
	• 9% absolute improvement in 3-year overall survival, mainly for those able to complete therapy
	• Delays in treatment and dose modifications because of toxicity are common
	• Often cannot be delivered as planned; outcomes for these patients are not known
Neoadjuvant chemotherapy	• Requires a functional multidisciplinary team and multidisciplinary consultation early in the management process
	• Hazard ratio for survival 0.86 (95% CI 0.77–0.95; $p = 0.003$)
	• 5% absolute improvement in 5-year overall survival (from 45% to 50%) with platinum-based regimens compared with radical cystectomy alone
	• Factors that predict benefit remain poorly defined
	• More likely to complete the planned course of therapy than for adjuvant therapy
	• Monitoring during treatment is essential to detect progressive disease early
	• Definitive surgery should be performed as soon as the acute toxicities of neoadjuvant therapy have resolved
	• Patients with pathological complete remission have better outcomes

CI, confidence interval.

Current recommendations supported by practice guidelines indicate the following.

- All patients with muscle-invasive bladder cancer (stage T2 or above) without distant metastases should be managed in a multidisciplinary setting.
- Patients considered suitable for systemic chemotherapy should be offered cisplatin-based neoadjuvant therapy.
- Adjuvant therapy should still be considered for patients requiring urgent surgical management.
- The strongest data relate to cisplatin-based chemotherapy regimens. Patients who are unfit for cisplatin may expect smaller benefits, which may influence decisions about whether perioperative therapy is appropriate.
- There is no evidence that further postoperative chemotherapy adds benefit for patients who still have viable tumor at cystectomy after preoperative chemotherapy.
- All suitable patients should be considered for clinical trials, if available and appropriate.

Multimodality and bladder-preserving therapy

Whilst radical cystectomy is the curative modality used for most patients with cancer that is clinically confined to the bladder, not all patients are medically suitable for this procedure, or choose not to undergo it. Medically unfit patients may derive better palliative benefit from more conservative therapy such as radiation therapy or best supportive care. Bladder-conserving definitive treatment can be considered for appropriate patients – generally those with smaller-volume cancers. This approach integrates systemic chemotherapy with radiation therapy, the former primarily acting as a radiosensitizer. Chemotherapy in combination with radiation therapy may also assist in eradicating micrometastatic disease; simpler regimens and lower doses are used compared with chemotherapy for overt metastatic disease. Finally, some patients may benefit from multimodality approaches combining two or more of surgery, radiation therapy and systemic treatment.

Unfortunately, there is no high-level evidence that compares bladder-preserving approaches and radical cystectomy. A large retrospective study of 348 patients with stage T2–T4a disease assessed outcomes after treatment with cisplatin and radiation therapy in the context of maximal transurethral resection of tumor, and neoadjuvant or adjuvant chemotherapy.[21] Patients were monitored with repeat biopsy, and subsequent treatment was guided by the initial tumor response. Patients experiencing complete remission received additional chemotherapy and a boost of radiation. Complete remission was observed in 72% of patients. Disease-specific and overall survival rates were excellent and comparable to contemporary cystectomy data. Cystectomy was required in 144 patients with suboptimal response or recurrent disease; no patient required cystectomy for treatment-related toxicity.

Current recommendations include combination chemoradiotherapy as a reasonable alternative to cystectomy for selected patients. Some patients may still require further therapy such as cystectomy for local control or palliation in the event of progression after bladder-preserving therapy, or intractable side effects of therapy such as urgency, frequency due to small bladder volume, hematuria or obstruction.

Various cytotoxic agents can be administered as radiosensitizers but the doses and schedules are different from conventional systemic therapy for advanced disease. The expected outcome is improvement in local control, rather than prevention or management of distant metastatic disease. The cytotoxic drugs most frequently used as radiosensitizers include cisplatin, docetaxel, paclitaxel, 5-fluorouracil (as monotherapy or with mitomycin) and capecitabine. Low-dose gemcitabine has also been used but can be associated with substantial toxicity from radiation, and other drugs are probably better alternatives. Carboplatin has also been used but is probably inferior to cisplatin as a radiosensitizer. Notably, patients receiving radiation therapy with palliative intent probably should not receive concurrent cytotoxic radiosensitizer treatment, as there is no evidence of improved palliative outcomes and the risk of toxicity is increased substantially.

Key points – treatment of muscle-invasive disease

- Bacillus Calmette–Guérin treatment is not indicated for bladder cancer that is T2 or higher.
- Surgical resection (radical or partial cystectomy) is the mainstay of treatment for patients suitable for surgery.
- Adequate node dissection should be performed at the time of cystectomy.
- For patients being managed with curative intent, chemoradiotherapy should be considered as an alternative to surgery, with appropriate multidisciplinary input.
- Cytotoxic drugs are used in the context of chemoradiotherapy with the intention of improving local disease control rather than achieving distant control.
- Toxicity is greater with combined chemotherapy and radiation than with radiation therapy alone.
- Patients treated with palliative intent are probably best offered radiation therapy only if surgery is not appropriate.

Key references

1. Chang SS, Boorjian SA, Chou R et al. Diagnosis and treatment of non-muscle invasive bladder cancer: AUA/SUO guideline. *J Urol* 2016;196:1021–9.

2. Herr HW, Bochner BH, Dalbagni G et al. Impact of the number of lymph nodes retrieved on outcome in patients with muscle invasive bladder cancer. *J Urol* 2002;167:1295–8.

3. Fleischmann A, Thalmann GN, Markwalder R, Studer UE. Extracapsular extension of pelvic lymph node metastases from urothelial carcinoma of the bladder is an independent prognostic factor. *J Clin Oncol* 2005;23:2358–65.

4. Koppie TM, Vickers AJ, Vora K et al. Standardization of pelvic lymphadenectomy performed at radical cystectomy: can we establish a minimum number of lymph nodes that should be removed? *Cancer* 2006;107:2368–74.

5. Leissner J, Ghoneim MA, Abol-Enein H et al. Extended radical lymphadenectomy in patients with urothelial bladder cancer: results of a prospective multicenter study. *J Urol* 2004;171:139–44.

6. Donat SM, Shabsigh A, Savage C et al. Potential impact of postoperative early complications on the timing of adjuvant chemotherapy in patients undergoing radical cystectomy: a high-volume tertiary cancer center experience. *Eur Urol* 2009;55:177–85.

7. Pang KH, Groves R, Venugopal S et al. Prospective implementation of enhanced recovery after surgery protocols to radical cystectomy. *Eur Urol* 2017; Aug 8 [Epub ahead of print; http://dx.doi.org/10.1016/j.eururo.2017.07.031].

8. Daneshmand S, Ahmadi H, Schuckman AK et al. Enhanced recovery protocol after radical cystectomy for bladder cancer. *J Urol* 2014;192:50–5.

9. Xu W, Daneshmand S, Bazargani ST et al. Postoperative pain management after radical cystectomy: comparing traditional versus enhanced recovery protocol pathway. *J Urol* 2015;194:1209–13.

10. Lee CT, Chang SS, Kamat AM et al. Alvimopan accelerates gastrointestinal recovery after radical cystectomy: a multicenter randomized placebo-controlled trial. *Eur Urol* 2014;66:265–72.

11. Gakis G, Efstathiou J, Lerner SP et al. ICUD-EAU International Consultation on Bladder Cancer 2012: radical cystectomy and bladder preservation for muscle-invasive urothelial carcinoma of the bladder. *Eur Urol* 2013;63:45–57.

12. Madeb R, Messing EM. Gender, racial and age differences in bladder cancer incidence and mortality. *Urol Oncol* 2004;22:86–92.

13. Karakiewicz PI, Shariat SF, Palapattu GS et al. Nomogram for predicting disease recurrence after radical cystectomy for transitional cell carcinoma of the bladder. *J Urol* 2006;176:1354–61; discussion 1361–2.

14. Shariat SF, Karakiewicz PI, Palapattu GS et al. Nomograms provide improved accuracy for predicting survival after radical cystectomy. *Clin Cancer Res* 2006;12:6663–76.

15. Gandaglia G, Karl A, Novara G et al. Perioperative and oncologic outcomes of robot-assisted vs. open radical cystectomy in bladder cancer patients: a comparison of two high-volume referral centers. *Eur J Surg Oncol* 2016;42:1736–43.

16. Smith AB, Raynor MC, Pruthi RS. Peri- and postoperative outcomes of robot-assisted radical cystectomy (RARC). *BJU Int* 2011;108:969–75.

17. Houédé N, Pourquier P, Beuzeboc P. Review of current neoadjuvant and adjuvant chemotherapy in muscle-invasive bladder cancer. *Eur Urol Suppl* 2011;10:e20–5.

18. Traboulsi SL, Kassouf W. A review of neoadjuvant and adjuvant chemotherapy for nonmetastatic muscle invasive bladder cancer. *Urol Pract* 2016;3:41–9.

19. Vale CL, Advanced Bladder Cancer Meta-analysis Collaboration. Adjuvant chemotherapy for invasive bladder cancer (individual patient data). *Cochrane Database Syst Rev* 2006;19;(2):CD006018.

20. Advanced Bladder Cancer Meta-analysis Collaboration. Neoadjuvant chemotherapy for invasive bladder cancer. *Cochrane Database Syst Rev* 2004;Apr 18;(2):CD005246.

21. Efstathiou JA, Spiegel DY, Shipley WU et al. Long-term outcomes of selective bladder preservation by combined-modality therapy for invasive bladder cancer: the MGH experience. *Eur Urol* 2012;61:705–11.

7 Management of advanced and metastatic disease

A core principle in the management of solid tumors is to consider control of both the primary and metastatic disease. Several clinical scenarios occur in bladder cancer.

- **Cancers that are clearly confined to the bladder** can potentially be cured if the primary tumor can be removed or ablated, through surgery, radiation therapy or multimodality approaches, and there is no metastatic disease; 5-year survival rates are about 70%.[1] Management of these cancers is discussed in chapter on 'Management of non-muscle-invasive disease'.

- **Locally advanced cancers and tumors that have spread to loco-regional lymph nodes** are associated with an increased risk of local relapse and a higher risk of micrometastatic disease at diagnosis. Five-year survival is about 35%. Lymph node involvement is identified through lymph node dissection or accurate imaging. The primary cancer may still be amenable to local therapy, and is potentially curable in the absence of distant metastases. Optimum systemic therapy with cisplatin-based chemotherapy is standard of care for patients with adequate renal function who are suitable for chemotherapy.

- **Cancers predominantly involving the bladder** but where there is small-volume overt metastatic disease are unlikely to be cured with currently available modalities; treatment is therefore palliative in intent, which must be clearly understood from the outset. Five-year survival for patients with metastatic disease is approximately 5%, although this varies depending on the bulk of disease, response to therapy and patient factors, including comorbidities. The mainstay of therapy is systemic treatment to control the progression of metastatic disease although management of the primary cancer may be necessary to alleviate symptoms and to prevent future complications such as pain, intractable hematuria and upper urinary tract obstruction. Surgery or radiation therapy may therefore be necessary for management of the primary tumor, and sometimes for management of metastatic disease.

- **Cancers where the bulk of disease is metastatic** are currently incurable; the intention of treatment is therefore palliative. Ablative local therapies such as surgery or radiation therapy should only be used to ameliorate current and potential issues that compromise quality of life.

All these strategies are predicated on whether the patient is able to tolerate the proposed treatment, and other factors such as comorbidities may require modification of the treatment plan. Treatment decisions usually require multidisciplinary input. A key component of such discussions should be whether participation in a clinical trial is possible and an appropriate option for the patient to consider.

This chapter summarizes current clinical recommendations for the systemic therapy of loco-regional advanced or metastatic disease. The treatment landscape and resulting recommendations are likely to change over the next few years as clinical trials are completed, particularly those of immunotherapies (see page 71).

Systemic therapy for metastatic bladder cancer

The activity of various cytotoxic drugs such as doxorubicin (Adriamycin), methotrexate, vinblastine and cisplatin against urothelial bladder cancer has been recognized since the 1970s. Response rates with cisplatin monotherapy were initially reported to be as high as 40%, although subsequent studies showed that response rates of 10–15% were more realistic. Other drugs such as paclitaxel and gemcitabine were also subsequently shown to have activity as monotherapies.

The first combination chemotherapy regimen to be widely used in clinical practice was cisplatin, methotrexate and vinblastine (CMV), which showed an overall response rate of 56% in a small single-arm study, half of which were complete remissions (notably in the era before computed tomography).[2] MVAC (methotrexate, vinblastine, doxorubicin and cisplatin) was shown to be superior to single-agent cisplatin for relevant endpoints of tumor response, duration of remission and overall survival (OS).[3] CMV and MVAC have been the mainstay of chemotherapy for metastatic urothelial bladder cancer for many years. Unfortunately, however, both regimens are difficult to deliver safely and are associated with substantial toxicity, including bone marrow suppression, neutropenic sepsis, mucositis, neuropathy, ototoxicity, nausea and vomiting, requiring frequent hospitalization, and sometimes leading to treatment-related death. These cytotoxic regimens can now be used in a broader range of patients since the development of supportive care measures such as antiemetics and colony-stimulating factors; previously, only the fittest patients were able to tolerate these cytotoxic regimens.

The treatment of metastatic bladder cancer was transformed following publication of a randomized Phase III trial comparing MVAC versus gemcitabine and cisplatin (GC).[4,5] The study was somewhat ambitiously designed to demonstrate a 33% improvement in OS with GC, rather than as an equivalence or non-inferiority study. The survival curves for the two regimens were similar, and the trial did not meet its primary endpoint. However, GC was found to be better tolerated than MVAC and was adopted as standard of care for the treatment of metastatic disease. GC has become the de facto standard for trials in other settings, even though this is not supported by high-level evidence. Modifications to the regimen are frequently made (often with little supporting evidence), such as splitting the dose of cisplatin, dropping treatment weeks or shortening treatment cycles, modifying the gemcitabine dosage, or substitution with drugs such as carboplatin. It is important to recognize when and how far we should go beyond high-level evidence when making treatment decisions with patients.

Improvements in supportive care have led to renewed interest in older chemotherapy combinations. One new approach is the intensification of treatment, such as accelerated[6] or high-dose MVAC, with granulocyte colony-stimulating factor support.[7] These regimens are generally much better tolerated than the original MVAC regimen and outcomes are at least comparable to those with GC, and perhaps numerically superior, although this has been difficult to prove statistically and remains controversial. Further modifications such as the addition of a taxane to GC increased the toxicity without substantially improving outcomes and therefore are not recommended. Chemotherapy regimens in common use for the first-line treatment of metastatic bladder cancer are summarized in Table 7.1.

TABLE 7.1

**Outcomes with chemotherapy regimens in common use
for the first-line treatment of metastatic bladder cancer**

Regimen	Response rate (% complete response)	Progression-free survival (months)	Overall survival (months)	Rate of grade 3/4 toxicity (%)	Death rate (%)
GC[4,5]	49 (12)	7.4	13.8	71	1
MVAC[3]	58 (11)	9.6	14	62	4
High dose MVAC/G-CSF[7]	64 (21)	9.5	15.1	20	3

GC, gemcitabine and cisplatin; G-CSF, granulocyte colony-stimulating factor;
MVAC, methotrexate, vinblastine, doxorubicin and cisplatin.

The dosing and scheduling details of cytotoxic chemotherapy regimens for advanced or metastatic bladder cancer are summarized in Table 7.2. Useful reviews of chemotherapy have been published by Yafi and colleagues[8] and Oing and colleagues.[9]

Recent clinical trials have targeted a so-called 'cisplatin-ineligible' population. The criteria for this designation are rather soft and can include:

- Eastern Cooperative Oncology Group performance status (PS) 2 or worse
- glomerular filtration rate (GFR) less than 60 mL/min
- pre-existing neuropathy or ototoxicity
- increased risk for neuropathy or ototoxicity (e.g. diabetes, alcohol misuse, occupational noise exposure)
- congestive cardiac failure or other inability to manage a fluid load.

However, not all these factors indicate unsuitability for cisplatin. Many 'cisplatin-ineligible' patients who enter trials have only one of these criteria, most commonly poor PS or reduced GFR, which means that many of these trials are not generalizable to real-world practice. While poor PS and reduced GFR are both relative contraindications to cisplatin, PS may be compromised by other conditions that will be unaffected by cisplatin, or may improve if symptoms are due to a tumor that subsequently responds to cisplatin. Patients with GFR of

TABLE 7.2

Chemotherapy regimens commonly used in all lines of treatment for metastatic bladder cancer

Drug	Regimen	Outcomes
Vinflunine[10]	320 mg/m² IV every 3 weeks (dose depending on performance status)	Response rate 9% Improvement in PFS but not OS
Carboplatin[11]	AUC 5 IV on day 1 every 3 weeks	Response rate 12%
Paclitaxel[12]	80 mg/m² IV weekly or 175 mg/m² IV over 3 hours every 3 weeks	Response rate 10–40%
Docetaxel[13]	75 mg/m² IV every 3 weeks	Response rate 30%
Pemetrexed[14]	500 mg/m² IV every 3 weeks (with vitamin B_{12} and folic acid prophylaxis)	Response rate 27% Median PFS 2.9 months Median OS 9.6 months
Nab-paclitaxel[15]	260 mg/m² IV every 3 weeks	Response rate 27.7%, almost all partial responses

AUC, area under the curve; IV, intravenous; Nab, nanoparticle albumin-bound; OS, overall survival; PFS, progression-free survival.

40–60 mL/min can often be managed safely by splitting the cisplatin dose over 2 weeks (although there is little evidence to support this approach). In addition, it may be possible to improve renal function through the use of percutaneous nephrostomy tubes or ureteric stents if hydronephrosis or hydroureter are contributory factors. These points need to be considered when deciding whether cisplatin is appropriate for a specific patient, and when designing clinical trials.

Second and subsequent lines of chemotherapy

Tumors that have progressed after first-line chemotherapy cannot be cured with chemotherapy, and response rates are typically lower than with first-line setting. It is important to reiterate at this stage that the intent of treatment is palliative, which can often be an uncomfortable conversation.

Chemotherapy may still be a reasonable palliative option as long as all other palliative objectives are addressed and quality of life is not impaired by treatment. The literature contains many examples of small studies in the post-first-line setting, for both cisplatin-eligible and cisplatin-ineligible patients. Response rates with active agents range from 20% to 80%. Use of complex regimens such as doublets or triplets does not seem to improve outcomes, and toxicity is substantially worse with combinations than with monotherapy. Patients who have had good responses previously may sometimes respond well to re-challenge with the same agents. Example regimens are shown in Table 7.2 (noting that not all drugs will be available in all regions).

General principles of treatment

The general principles of chemotherapy for advanced or metastatic disease are summarized in Table 7.3.

Palliation and best supportive care

Patients with incurable disease must be managed with palliative intent. Any treatment must provide some possibility of benefit, and this benefit should outweigh the predicted risks. Early involvement of a broad multidisciplinary management team is important and should include palliative care, nursing and allied health professionals.

Active treatment may still be appropriate, particularly if symptoms are amenable to such therapies and the patient is well enough to tolerate them. It is therefore reasonable to consider surgery, radiation therapy, cytotoxic chemotherapy or other active approaches within the context of supportive care and palliative intent. Practitioners delivering these therapies must be experienced and fully aware of the benefits and limitations of what they offer, bearing in mind the wellbeing of the patient and their broader social situation, including effects on family and carers. The financial implications of treatment may also require consideration.

TABLE 7.3

General principles of chemotherapy for advanced or metastatic disease

• Patient selection is paramount, although newer regimens and improvements in supportive care have made chemotherapy more tolerable for more patients.

• GC remains the standard of care. Variants such as dose-dense MVAC are acceptable alternatives, although there is no high-level evidence to confirm this.

• Other drug combinations remain experimental. Addition of agents generally increases the toxicity but without substantial improvement in response or survival outcomes.

• Carboplatin is inferior to cisplatin and should not be substituted in combination regimens. Patients who are medically unfit to receive cisplatin should receive individualized treatment with palliative intent. Any active and tolerable monotherapy is a reasonable alternative for these patients.

• Evidence to support the use of cytotoxic chemotherapy after first-line treatment is weak. Combination regimens are probably not justified and monotherapies are preferable.

• Clinical trials may be an option for some patients, including those with contraindications to cisplatin, poor PS or comorbidities.

• The palliative intent of treatment should be explained at the outset. Early referral for palliative and other supportive care resources should be considered. Multidisciplinary input is key.

• Patients with tumors of non-urothelial histology are largely excluded from trials so the evidence base for use of chemotherapy in these patients is weak.

GC, gemcitabine and cisplatin; MVAC, methotrexate, vinblastine, doxorubicin and cisplatin; PS, performance status.

Many symptoms can be treated with simple and non-invasive measures, for example:

- optimal pain management, possibly involving a specialist pain management team
- detection and management of urinary tract infections
- modification of other treatments (such as cessation of antiplatelet drugs in a patient with intractable hematuria)
- blood transfusion (with defined stopping points)
- radiation therapy for symptomatic metastatic disease
- management of other symptoms of metastatic disease.

Key points – management of advanced and metastatic disease

- Management of patients with advanced or metastatic disease is complex and requires a multidisciplinary approach.
- Management of both local and distant metastatic disease should be considered.
- The intent of treatment for patients with metastatic disease is optimal palliation (improved quality of life with or without prolonging survival). The benefits of any treatment must outweigh the risks.
- Perioperative chemotherapy should be considered for suitable patients with high-risk bladder-confined disease, but preoperative chemotherapy is preferred where possible.
- Combination chemoradiotherapy can be an alternative to cystectomy for the management of locally advanced disease.
- Cisplatin-based chemotherapy can provide excellent outcomes for some patients with advanced or metastatic disease.
- Radiation therapy to the primary or appropriate metastatic sites can provide useful palliation.
- Combination chemoradiotherapy to the bladder is best reserved for patients being treated with curative intent.

Key references

1. Siegel RL, Miller KD, Jemal A. Cancer statistics, 2018. *CA Cancer J Clin* 2018;68:7–30.

2. Harker WG, Meyers FJ, Freiha FS et al. Cisplatin, methotrexate, and vinblastine (CMV): an effective chemotherapy regimen for metastatic transitional cell carcinoma of the urinary tract. A Northern California Oncology Group study. *J Clin Oncol* 1985;3:1463–70.

3. Loehrer PJ, Sr., Einhorn LH, Elson PJ et al. A randomized comparison of cisplatin alone or in combination with methotrexate, vinblastine, and doxorubicin in patients with metastatic urothelial carcinoma: a cooperative group study. *J Clin Oncol* 1992;10:1066–73.

4. von der Maase H, Hansen SW, Roberts JT et al. Gemcitabine and cisplatin versus methotrexate, vinblastine, doxorubicin, and cisplatin in advanced or metastatic bladder cancer: results of a large, randomized, multinational, multicenter, phase III study. *J Clin Oncol* 2000;18:3068–77.

5. von der Maase H, Sengelov L, Roberts JT et al. Long-term survival results of a randomized trial comparing gemcitabine plus cisplatin, with methotrexate, vinblastine, doxorubicin, plus cisplatin in patients with bladder cancer. *J Clin Oncol* 2005;23:4602–8.

6. Edeline J, Loriot Y, Culine S et al. Accelerated MVAC chemotherapy in patients with advanced bladder cancer previously treated with a platinum-gemcitabine regimen. *Eur J Cancer* 2012;48:114–6.

7. Sternberg CN, de Mulder PH, Schornagel JH et al. Randomized phase III trial of high-dose-intensity methotrexate, vinblastine, doxorubicin, and cisplatin (MVAC) chemotherapy and recombinant human granulocyte colony-stimulating factor versus classic MVAC in advanced urothelial tract tumors: European Organisation for Research and Treatment of Cancer protocol no. 30924. *J Clin Oncol* 2001;19:2638–46.

8. Yafi FA, North S, Kassouf W. First- and second-line therapy for metastatic urothelial carcinoma of the bladder. *Curr Oncol* 2011;18:e25–34.

9. Oing C, Rink M, Oechsle K et al. Second line chemotherapy for advanced and metastatic urothelial carcinoma: Vinflunine and beyond – a comprehensive review of the current literature. *J Urol* 2016;195:254–63.

10. Bellmunt J, Theodore C, Demkov T et al. Phase III trial of vinflunine plus best supportive care compared with best supportive care alone after a platinum-containing regimen in patients with advanced transitional cell carcinoma of the urothelial tract. *J Clin Oncol* 2009;27:4454–61.

11. Waxman J, Barton C. Carboplatin-based chemotherapy for bladder cancer. *Cancer Treat Rev* 1993;19(Suppl C):21–5.

12. Vaughn DJ, Broome CM, Hussain M et al. Phase II trial of weekly paclitaxel in patients with previously treated advanced urothelial cancer. *J Clin Oncol* 2002;20:937–40.

13. McCaffrey JA, Hilton S, Mazumdar M et al. Phase II trial of docetaxel in patients with advanced or metastatic transitional-cell carcinoma. *J Clin Oncol* 1997;15:1853–7.

14. Sweeney CJ, Roth BJ, Kabbinavar FF et al. Phase II study of pemetrexed for second-line treatment of transitional cell cancer of the urothelium. *J Clin Oncol* 2006;24:3451–7.

15. Ko YJ, Canil CM, Mukherjee SD et al. Nanoparticle albumin-bound paclitaxel for second-line treatment of metastatic urothelial carcinoma: a single group, multicentre, phase 2 study. *Lancet Oncol* 2013;14:769–76.

Bladder cancer has long been considered responsive to immunological manipulation. Treatment of non-muscle-invasive urothelial bladder cancer with bacillus Calmette–Guérin is well established as standard of care, see pages 45–48.

After decades with few clinical trials or advances in treatment, recent years have seen the advent of new and efficacious immunotherapeutic approaches, and several new treatments have been approved, across all stages of urothelial cancer. The field has suddenly become both crowded and exciting. This chapter provides a snapshot as at early 2018; however, substantial changes in practice are likely as new information continues to emerge.

Principles of immunotherapy

The principles of effective immunotherapy for solid tumors have been extensively reviewed.[1-3] The key points are as follows.

- Tumor cells express antigens that provide variable levels of distinction from normal tissues.
- These antigens are taken up and processed by antigen-presenting cells such as dendritic cells.
- Processed antigen is then presented to cells of the immune system, including T and B cells.
- The immune system recognizes and responds to these antigens, particularly through the development of cytotoxic T cell antigen-specific responses and development of immunologic memory.
- Cytotoxic effector T cells migrate to the site of the cancer and attack cells expressing the antigen.

These processes evolved to facilitate recognition of intracellular pathogens such as viruses, and the immune system uses the same processes to recognize and eliminate tumor cells. Many tumor cells are eliminated before clinical evidence of cancer emerges, and some tumors live in equilibrium with the immune system until another event disturbs this equilibrium in one direction or the other. However, tumor cells adapt and evolve through natural selection to evade the immune system. Clinically apparent cancers are ones that, by definition, have evaded immune recognition or elimination. Our growing understanding of the processes and mechanisms underlying immune processes has led to new approaches to manipulation of the responses. Key control points in this process that can be manipulated are illustrated in Figure 8.1 and described in Table 8.1. Drugs targeting many of these molecules and processes are in development, as monotherapies and in combination with other immunomodulators or chemotherapeutic agents.

Blockade of CTLA-4 (cytotoxic T-lymphocyte-associated protein 4) was one of the first effective systemic immunotherapy approaches in the modern era. CTLA-4 mediates inhibitory signals to the T cell during its interaction with antigen-presenting cells such as dendritic cells, ensuring that the immune system does not become overactivated in an uncontrolled fashion. Monoclonal antibodies against CTLA-4,

TABLE 8.1

Tumor characteristics required for effective immunotherapy

Inherent to tumor	'Mutational and neoantigen load' of the cancer
	Presence of microsatellite instability
	Presence of other DNA repair deficiencies
	Epigenetic regulation of antigen expression*
Immunologic context	*PD-L1 expression*
	Immune priming and/or boosting
	'Permissive' microenvironment to enable effective killing
	Inflammatory genetic signature
	Absence of immunosuppression
Factors missing or uncertain in urothelial cancer	Viral antigens
	Variability of tumor-infiltrating lymphocytes

*Italic indicates potentially modifiable factors that may affect the responsiveness of a tumor to treatment. PD-L1, programmed cell death ligand 1.

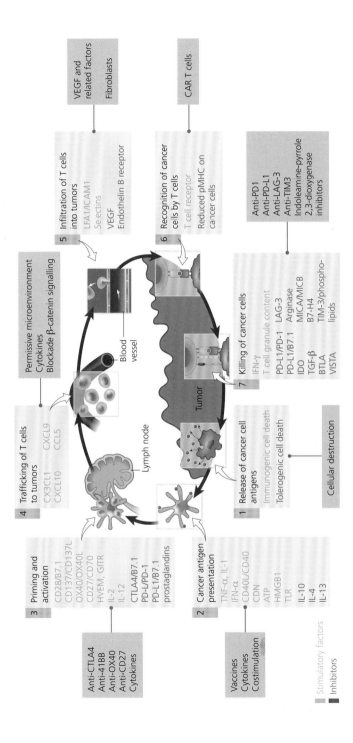

Figure 8.1 The cancer immunity cycle and potential approaches for therapeutic manipulation. Reproduced from Chen & Mellman[4] with permission. CAR, chimeric antigen receptor; CTLA-4, cytotoxic T-lymphocyte-associated protein 4; IDO, indoleamine-pyrrole 2,3-dioxygenase; PD-1, programmed cell death protein 1; PD-L1, PD ligand 1; VEGF, vascular endothelial growth factor.

such as ipilimumab and tremelimumab, are approved or are being developed for a range of indications. The programmed cell death protein 1 (PD-1) axis has also been a key target, described in more detail below. Simultaneous blockade of both CTLA-4 and the PD-1 axis is a logical approach and in some settings improves clinical outcomes but increases the risk of significant autoimmune toxicities.

It is important to remember that immunotherapy does not directly target the biology of the cancer; the intention is to activate or 'de-repress' the normal immune system. These approaches should therefore, in theory, be applicable to virtually any type of malignancy. Indeed, the clinical development of these agents has been rapid, with evidence of activity across many tumor types. However, not every tumor type responds, and not every patient with a potentially responsive cancer will benefit. It is not yet possible to predict reliably who will or will not respond to these agents.

PD-1 axis

Clinical development in bladder cancer is currently focusing on agents that interfere with the PD-1 axis, particularly the PD-1 receptor and its ligand (PD-L1). PD-1 is a cell surface 'checkpoint' that has an important role in regulating the recruitment and activation of T cells. Overexpression of this receptor by tumor cells has been reported in several solid tumors, including bladder cancer. Binding of PD-L1 to the PD-1 receptor affects the immune response to cancer cells in two ways.

- In the lymph nodes, overexpression of PD-L1 in tumor-infiltrating immune cells can prevent the priming and activation of new cytotoxic T cells, and subsequently prevent recruitment of these immune cells to the tumor.
- Within the tumor microenvironment, up-regulation of PD-L1 on dendritic cells leads to deactivation of cytotoxic T cells.

In both cases, binding of PD-L1 to PD-1 on the surface of T cells results in the development of T-cell tolerance, with reduced T-cell proliferation, decreased cytokine expression and impaired antigen recognition (Figure 8.2).

Blockade of the PD-1 axis removes the inhibition of effector T cells, promoting cellular cytotoxicity (Figure 8.3). Expression of PD-1 is low in non-cancerous tissue so the effects of PD-1 are largely confined to the tumor site. Furthermore, therapies that act on PD-1 have the

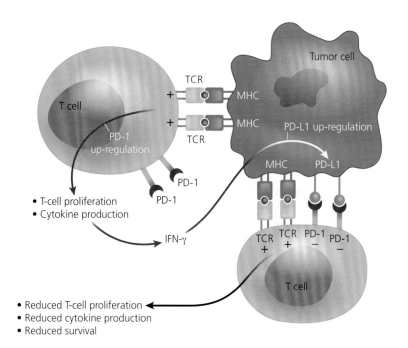

Figure 8.2 Effects of the programmed cell death protein 1 (PD-1) receptor on T-cell function. Binding of PD-1 on the surface of T cells to its ligand (PD-L1) on tumor cells leads to the development of T-cell tolerance, with reduced T-cell proliferation, decreased cytokine expression and impaired antigen recognition. IFN, interferon; MHC, major histocompatibility complex; TCR, T-cell receptor. Adapted from Buchbinder & Desai, 2016.[5]

potential to reset tumor-related alterations in the immune system while leaving normal peripheral tolerance to self-antigens unaffected. Many monoclonal antibodies have been developed against PD-1 (e.g. nivolumab, pembrolizumab) and PD-L1 (e.g. atezolizumab, avelumab, durvalumab) and others are in development.

PD-1-targeted immunotherapies
The first PD-1-targeted immunotherapy to be approved was atezolizumab, based on results from the Phase II IMvigor 210 trial, which showed an overall response rate of 15% and acceptable toxicity.

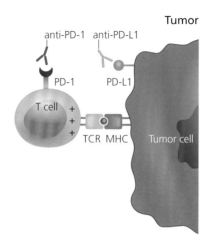

Figure 8.3 Mechanism of action of the PD-1 and PD-L1 inhibitors. MHC, major histocompatability complex; PD-1, programmed cell death protein 1; PD-L1, programmed cell death ligand 1; TCR, T-cell receptor. Adapted from Bellmunt et al., 2017[6]

At the time of writing, five monoclonal antibodies targeting either PD-1 or PD-L1 have been approved by the US Food and Drug Administration (FDA) for the management of advanced or metastatic urothelial cancer (Table 8.2). All received breakthrough therapy designation and were approved via priority review, based on data from Phase II single-arm studies, with the exception of pembrolizumab, which was compared with chemotherapy (investigators' choice). Note that the outcomes of further trials may affect approval and subsequent use of these agents.

Table 8.3 summarizes key data from trials for the five PD-1 axis inhibitors. Some common themes have emerged.
- Response rates are about 20% with single agents.
- Occasionally patients demonstrate remarkable responses, which can be prolonged.
- Monotherapy with these agents is generally well tolerated, with a low incidence of severe immune-related adverse events.
- Responses cannot be reliably predicted using existing tissue-based assays of PD-L1 or other available markers.

The most convincing data so far relate to pembrolizumab, which is the first product for which Phase III results were reported. The Keynote-045 Phase III trial demonstrated that pembrolizumab was active in the second-line setting for patients whose cancers had progressed after cisplatin-based chemotherapy, and provided a significant overall survival (OS) benefit compared with standard

TABLE 8.2

Monoclonal antibodies targeting the PD-1 axis approved by the US Food and Drug Administration for the treatment of advanced or metastatic bladder cancer

Mechanism	Drug	Date approved	Indication*
PD-1 inhibitor	Nivolumab (Opdivo®; Bristol-Myers Squibb)	Feb 2017	Locally advanced or metastatic urothelial carcinoma that has progressed during or following platinum-containing chemotherapy, or within 12 months of neoadjuvant or adjuvant platinum-containing chemotherapy
	Pembrolizumab (Keytruda®; Merck)	May 2017	
PD-L1 inhibitor	Atezolizumab (Tecentriq®; Genetech)	May 2016	
	Avelumab (Bavencio®; EMD Serono)	May 2017	
	Durvalumab (Imfinzi®; AstraZeneca)	May 2017	

*Atezolizumab and pembrolizumab are also approved for the first-line treatment of locally advanced or metastatic urothelial carcinoma in patients not eligible for cisplatin-containing chemotherapy.
PD-1, programmed cell death protein 1; PD-L1, programmed cell death ligand 1.

chemotherapy: 10.3 versus 7.4 months (hazard ratio for death 0.73, 95% confidence interval [CI] 0.59–0.91; $p = 0.002$).[7]

Other drugs in this class are likely to have similar efficacy, as illustrated in Table 8.3. However, study design needs to be considered carefully when looking at trial results. For example, the IMvigor 211 trial, which compared atezolizumab versus chemotherapy following failure of platinum-based chemotherapy, did not meet its OS primary endpoint,[8] although this was probably because of the way the statistical analysis was planned, and overconfidence in the PD-L1 tissue assay: the outcome was negative for the apparently PD-L1-

TABLE 8.3

Key data from trials of PD-1-targeted agents in the second-line treatment of urothelial cancer

Drug (target)	Trial (no. evaluable patients)	Phase	Overall response rate	PFS (months)	Other endpoints
Nivolumab (PD-1)	CheckMate 275[9] (n = 270)	II	20% (53 responses: 7 CR; 46 PR)	2.0	Estimated median DOR: 10.3 months at data cut-off
Pembrolizumab (PD-1)	Keynote-045[7] (n = 542)	III	21% (vs 11% with CT)	2.1 (vs 3.3 with CT)	DOR: 1.6+ to 15.6+ months vs 4.3 with CT OS: 10.3 vs 7.4 months (p = 0.002)
Atezolizumab (PD-L1)	IMvigor 210[10] (n = 316)	II	15%	2.1	
	IMvigor 211[8] (n = 931)	III	OS endpoint not reached		
Avelumab (PD-L1)	JAVELIN[11] (n = 249)	Ib	17% (n = 161 with ≥ 6 months' data; 9 CR: 18 PR)	6.3 weeks	Median DOR not reached (95% CI 42.1 weeks to not estimable) Median OS 6.5 months
Durvalumab (PD-L1)	Study 1108[12] (n = 182)	I/II	17.6%	1.5	OS 18.2 months at data cut-off

All studies except Keynote-045 and IMvigor 211 were single arm.
CI, confidence interval; CR, complete response; CT, chemotherapy; DOR, duration of response; OS, overall survival; PD-1, programmed cell death protein 1; PD-L1, programmed cell death ligand 1; PFS, progression-free survival; PR, partial response.

expressing subset but positive when the entire study population was included.

Prediction of response

The identification of biomarkers, and therefore tests, that predict response to treatment has not been a priority in pharmaceutical drug development. This is changing with the development of immunotherapies and the pressure to be able to identify patients who are likely to benefit from treatment with particular monoclonal antibodies, such as trastuzumab in HER2-overexpressing breast cancer and *BRAF* mutations in melanoma. Availability of such validated tests would allow rational use of the drugs and avoid exposing patients to the adverse effects of drugs that might provide no clinical benefit. However, BRAF and HER2 are 'driver' molecules and their status can be accurately determined, whereas this is not the case with PD-L1.

Expression of PD-L1 is often associated with poorer outcomes in bladder cancer, regardless of the treatment used. It is logical to expect that expression of PD-L1 by tumor, immune or other cells in the tumor deposit would predict response to therapies targeted at the PD-1 axis; however, this has not yet been reliably shown to be the case, mainly because of deficiencies and variability in the available tissue-based assays for PD-L1.

For example, the Phase II IMvigor 210 study of atezolizumab (on which FDA approval was based) reported that 26% of patients who were classified as 'positive' for PD-L1 expression experienced a response, compared with 9.5% of participants classified as 'negative'. The FDA simultaneously approved the Ventana PD-L1 (SP142) assay to detect PD-L1 protein expression levels on patients' tumor-infiltrating immune cells to help physicians determine which patients may benefit most from treatment with atezolizumab.[13] However, the subsequent Phase III IMvigor 211 study did not confirm these findings.

The single-arm Phase I/II Study 1108 of durvalumab, which included 182 patients with locally advanced or metastatic urothelial carcinoma who experienced disease progression following platinum-containing chemotherapy, reported objective response rates (ORR) of 27.4% (95% CI 18.7–37.5) among the 95 patients with high PD-L1 expression, compared with 4.1% (95% CI 0.9–11.5) in the cohort of

73 patients with low or no PD-L1 expression.[12,14] The ORR in the overall population was 17.6% (95% CI 12.3–23.9).

The companion diagnostic was approved by the FDA simultaneously with durvalumab. However, the FDA labels for atezolizumab and durvalumab do not specify a requirement for PD-L1 testing, which is in contrast to other targeted drugs such as the BRAF inhibitors for use in melanoma, or indeed pembrolizumab in the treatment of gastric cancer. This lack of requirement to demonstrate PD-L1 expression implies a more widespread understanding of the lack of value of this test. In contrast, the FDA recently approved pembrolizumab as a 'tissue-agnostic', for cancers with microsatellite instability or DNA mismatch repair defects. This is the first time that the indication for an immunotherapy has been defined according to prior treatment and a set of molecular markers rather than the histological tissue of origin.

Variation in PD-L1 expression. Importantly, PD-L1 expression is both dynamic and sporadic: it probably changes over short periods, and PD-L1 is not necessarily expressed by all cells. It is therefore not surprising that measurement of PD-L1 expression in a small sample of tissue, perhaps obtained many years previously and stored under suboptimal conditions, does not correlate well with the probability of response to PD-1 axis blockade. Tissue PD-L1 expression has reasonable positive predictive value, in that cancers that are positive for PD-L1 expression are generally more likely to respond to PD-1-targeted therapies. However, cancers that do not appear to express PD-L1 may still respond to therapies targeted at the PD-1 axis.

Negative predictive value. Poor negative predictive value is probably more important but there is no test with adequate negative predictive value to inform clinicians that a specific patient is unlikely to respond to this immunotherapy and therefore should not be exposed to the risk of adverse effects with little hope of therapeutic benefit, but instead should have another treatment such as chemotherapy.

First-line studies
Atezolizumab was approved by the FDA in April 2017 for the first-line treatment of 'cisplatin-ineligible' patients with locally advanced or

metastatic bladder cancer. This approval was based on data from a cohort of 119 patients in the Imvigor 210 trial. The ORR was 23.5%, including a complete response rate of 36.7%. Median progression-free survival was 2.7 months (95% CI 2.1–4.2), and median OS was 15.9 months (95% CI 10.4 to not estimable).[15]

The Keynote-052 Phase II trial examined the activity of pembrolizumab as first-line treatment in 'cisplatin-ineligible' patients. Pembrolizumab showed activity in this group, of which fewer than half were probably truly cisplatin-ineligible but who probably represented the least fit of the treatment-naïve population.

As yet, there are insufficient data to recommend the routine use of immunotherapy instead of cisplatin-based chemotherapy as first-line therapy, although this question is currently being addressed in several clinical trials. Pembrolizumab may be a reasonable alternative for first-line therapy in less-fit and cisplatin-ineligible patients. Avelumab, nivolumab and durvalumab are also being evaluated in the first-line setting.

Adverse effects of immunotherapy

The main adverse effects of immunotherapy relate to autoimmunity, that is, unmasking of immune responses against normal tissues. The systems most commonly affected are the skin, gastrointestinal tract, liver, endocrine system (including hypophysitis) and respiratory tract. However, rarer effects can occur, such as neurological or myocardial autoimmunity. Patients need to be treated by teams experienced in the management of these effects, and should be fully informed so that subtle autoimmunity can be detected and treated before significant toxicity occurs. Examples include endocrine dysfunction (panhypopituitarism, hypothyroidism, hypogonadism, hypoadrenalism), which can be subtle in presentation and easily missed but which can become life-threatening. Similarly, mild diarrhea may result from autoimmune colitis but without treatment can deteriorate and become fatal. Immune-related adverse events can usually be managed according to algorithms for immunosuppression, although some patients may not recover and may need ongoing management such as hormone replacement therapy. Interestingly, autoimmunity is correlated with an increased probability of an anticancer benefit but treatment of autoimmunity does not abrogate the antitumor effect. The reasons for this discrepancy remain unclear.

Key points – immunotherapy

- Five immunotherapies have recently been approved for the second-line treatment of advanced or metastatic bladder cancer, and two have also been approved in the first-line setting.
- There is good evidence that second-line treatment after cisplatin-based chemotherapy is generally well tolerated, efficacious, and can confer a survival advantage.
- First-line treatment is also efficacious, particularly in patients less likely to tolerate cytotoxic chemotherapy.
- So far there is no strong evidence that immunotherapies targeted at the programmed cell death protein 1 (PD-1) axis differ substantially in terms of efficacy or toxicity.
- A survival benefit has been shown with pembrolizumab versus chemotherapy but not atezolizumab (likely a reflection of the study design); however, survival data from the trials of the other immunotherapies are not yet mature.
- Combination strategies are being explored; these may be more active than monotherapies but are likely to be more toxic and more costly.
- Current tissue-based programmed cell death ligand 1 (PD-L1) assays do not reliably predict response or lack of response to PD-1-targeted therapy.
- The management of advanced and metastatic bladder cancer will evolve as the results of further trials emerge.

Key references

1. Aragon-Ching JB. Challenges and advances in the diagnosis, biology, and treatment of urothelial upper tract and bladder carcinomas. *Urol Oncol* 2017;35:462–4.

2. Funt SA, Rosenberg JE. Systemic, perioperative management of muscle-invasive bladder cancer and future horizons. *Nat Rev Clin Oncol* 2017;14:221–34.

3. Powles T, Smith K, Stenzl A, Bedke J. Immune checkpoint inhibition in metastatic urothelial cancer. *Eur Urol* 2017;72:477–81.

4. Chen DS, Mellman I. Oncology meets immunology: the cancer-immunity cycle. *Immunity* 2013;39: 1–10.

5. Buchbinder EI, Desai A. CTLA-4 and PD-1 pathways: similarities, differences, and implications of their inhibition. *Am J Clin Oncol* 2016;39:98–106.

6. Bellmunt J, Powles T, Vogelzang NJ. A review on the evolution of PD-1/PD-L1 immunotherapy for bladder cancer: the future is now. *Cancer Treat Rev* 2017;54:58–67.

7. Bellmunt J, de Wit R, Vaughn DJ et al. Pembrolizumab as second-line therapy for advanced urothelial carcinoma. *N Engl J Med* 2017;376:1015–26.

8. Powles T, Duran I, van der Heijden MS et al. Atezolizumab versus chemotherapy in patients with platinum-treated locally advanced or metastatic urothelial carcinoma (IMvigor211): a multicentre, open-label, phase 3 randomised controlled trial. *Lancet* 2017; Dec 18 [Epub ahead of print; http://dx.doi.org/10.1016/S0140-6736(17)33297-X].

9. Sharma P, Retz M, Siefker-Radtke A et al. Nivolumab in metastatic urothelial carcinoma after platinum therapy (CheckMate 275): a multicentre, single-arm, phase 2 trial. *Lancet Oncol* 2017;18:312–22.

10. Perez-Gracia JL, Loriot Y, Rosenberg JE et al. Atezolizumab in platinum-treated locally advanced or metastatic urothelial carcinoma: outcomes by prior number of regimens. *Eur Urol* 2017; Dec 19 [Epub ahead of print].

11. Patel MR, Ellerton J, Infante JR et al. Avelumab in metastatic urothelial carcinoma after platinum failure (JAVELIN Solid Tumor): pooled results from two expansion cohorts of an open-label, phase 1 trial. *Lancet Oncol* 2018;19:51–64.

12. Powles T, O'Donnell PH, Massard C et al. Efficacy and safety of durvalumab in locally advanced or metastatic urothelial carcinoma. *JAMA Oncol* 2017;14;3(9):e172411 [doi: 10.1001/jamaoncol.2017.2411].

13. FDA. FDA approves new, targeted treatment for bladder cancer. 2016. www.fda.gov/NewsEvents/Newsroom/PressAnnouncements/ucm501762.htm. Last accessed 30 January 2018.

14. FDA. Durvalumab (Imfinzi). 2017. www.fda.gov/Drugs/InformationOnDrugs/ApprovedDrugs/ucm555930.htm. Last accessed 30 January 2018.

15. Balar AV, Galsky MD, Rosenberg JE et al. Atezolizumab as first-line treatment in cisplatin-ineligible patients with locally advanced and metastatic urothelial carcinoma: a single-arm, multicentre, phase 2 trial. *Lancet* 2017;389:67–76.

9 Future trends

The mortality and morbidity of bladder cancer could be reduced in several ways:
- improving prevention
- earlier diagnosis
- better treatment of high-risk non-muscle-invasive disease
- improved use of existing therapies
- identification of biomarkers that allow better risk stratification and selection of treatment
- development of new therapies and rational combinations
- better involvement of palliative and supportive care.

Improving prevention

Smoking remains by far the most important contributor to the burden of bladder cancer around the world (see page 9). In fact, the link between smoking and bladder cancer is stronger than the link with lung cancer but is less well understood by the general population. Smoking is also the factor most amenable to modification through changes to individual behavior and public health measures. This requires changes to societal norms to make smoking an unacceptable behavior. Health authorities in many countries are introducing legislation that restricts where people can smoke, and programs that aim to reduce the uptake of smoking, particularly in younger people, and assisting smokers to quit. For example, in the UK smoking rates among young adults decreased from 26% in 2010 to 19% in 2016, and the number of adult smokers decreased from 17.2% in 2015 to 15.8% in 2016.[1]

Consideration must also be given to reducing incidental or sidestream (passive) exposure to smoke, particularly for those who cannot choose to avoid it, such as children, and workers in the hospitality industries. Legislation to ban smoking in public places and in the presence of children is being implemented in many countries. These measures will address numerous other health issues and are an extremely logical use of public healthcare expenditure.

Occupational exposure to carcinogens is now uncommon. Schistosomiasis remains a significant factor in bladder carcinogenesis in certain regions, although rates have fallen significantly over the last 25 years as measures to control schistosomiasis have been implemented.[2]

Earlier diagnosis

Bladder cancer is often a 'forgotten' cancer in the community, even though it is reported to be the most expensive cancer from diagnosis to death overall, accounting for substantial healthcare costs and resource use.[3]

As discussed in the 'Clinical Presentation' chapter, a key problem is that symptoms may be overlooked or ignored by the patient and physician, increasing the probability of disease being advanced at diagnosis. For example, a survey of more than 9600 people in five European countries found that 62% did not know the signs and symptoms of bladder cancer.[4] Improved public awareness of the symptoms of bladder cancer is therefore needed to allow earlier detection, when cure may be possible. One example is the 'blood in your pee' public awareness advertising in the UK (part of a larger 'Be clear on cancer' campaign by the National Health Service) and in Australia. It is also important that clinicians understand the importance of following up any incidence of hematuria (see page 27).

Current diagnostic modalities are invasive (cystoscopy) or have suboptimal sensitivity and/or specificity (urine cytology or other urine-based diagnostics) or are too costly for routine use. Innovative models such as 'one stop' clinics for evaluation of hematuria and performance of cystoscopy may improve outcomes (see page 31).

Tests for tumor markers that may reduce the use of cystoscopy are being explored (see page 33–35).

Better treatment of high-risk non-muscle-invasive disease

Most non-muscle-invasive bladder cancer is low or intermediate risk (low-grade Ta), can be managed endoscopically and requires only limited further assessment or treatment. High-risk disease (all Ta, T1, high-grade carcinoma in situ [CIS], or large volume Ta) is less common but accounts for the majority of health resources in this therapy area, in managing the initial disease and reducing the risk of recurrence or progression to more advanced or metastatic disease. Newer surgical and other ablative techniques, and enhanced endoscopic imaging with fluorescence cystoscopy, optical coherence tomography and confocal laser,[5] may improve diagnostic risk stratification and the definitive treatment of early disease. Standardization of protocols for adjunctive therapies such as bacillus Calmette–Guérin (BCG) treatment will also reduce the number of non-muscle-invasive cancers that progress to fatal invasive cancers. Hayne and colleagues have summarized the current status of several relevant trials with BCG.[6]

Advances in the near future will probably include systemic immunotherapy, if these treatments are shown to improve control or cure and reduce recurrence and progression, with an acceptable safety profile and cost-effectiveness. Treatment is also likely to be stratified according to molecular and genomic profiling of the tumor rather than conventional light microscopic appearance. More accurate imaging modalities may allow better detection and management of residual or micrometastatic disease, with consequent improvements in the stratification of patients into more appropriate treatment pathways.

Improved use of existing therapies

This has been the main focus of work to date, and considerable progress has been made across all stages of bladder cancer. Two surgical trials testing the potential benefit of extended pelvic and iliac lymphadenectomy at the time of radical cystectomy will define the optimal anatomic limits of this surgery.[7,8] Radiation therapy can be administered more safely at higher doses and with fewer side effects. Cytotoxic chemotherapy can now be safely delivered to many patients and previous definitions of cisplatin-ineligibility have been relaxed. These changes mean that treatment can be given more safely, at more effective doses, for the planned duration, and to a broader range of patients. Many patients now have excellent outcomes with established treatments such as systemic cytotoxic chemotherapy and further improvements could be realized through more widespread use of neoadjuvant chemotherapy for suitable patients.

Future advances in this area will be based on:

- better understanding of the biology of bladder cancer and consequent treatment selection, such as the identification of biomarkers that reliably predict who should receive immunotherapy instead of chemotherapy and markers that would point to a higher probability of response in subsequent lines of therapy
- high-level evidence of meaningful clinical benefit, particularly improved survival and quality of life, which have yet to be reported from early trials of immunotherapies
- rational combinations of existing therapy, such as chemotherapy and immunotherapy, or integration of small-molecule kinase inhibitors, possibly in selected patients based on characterization of tumor biology
- use of active therapies at earlier stages in the treatment pathways
- better access to therapies, particularly in low- or middle-income countries.

Identification of biomarkers that allow better risk stratification and treatment selection

Several relevant biomarkers for risk stratification and prediction of response to treatment of bladder cancer are being explored (e.g. FGFR, VEGFR, HER2, circulating tumor DNA) and some (e.g. PD-L1) are beginning to be used in clinical practice in the hope that this might increase the probability that patients receiving treatments aimed at such targets will respond to them; however, uptake of such assays remains limited on a global scale and it is not yet clear whether their use improves outcomes. Improvements in the specificity and sensitivity of assays are required before these approaches are used in routine practice.

Better technology in this arena, including tests that are less invasive than cystoscopy or biopsy and therefore more acceptable to patients, will lead to earlier diagnosis and treatment and reduction of costs. Future developments are likely to involve refinements based on rational assessment of the tumor biology based on genomic, proteomic or immunologic profiling. However, incorporation of these assays into clinical practice requires care, particularly if the tissue was not obtained recently (e.g. past cystectomy) or is not representative of the cancer (e.g. small endoscopic biopsy of a bladder tumor in a patient with widespread metastatic disease). We will do well to learn from experience with the PD-L1 assays and the effects that blind faith in an unproven biomarker can have on clinical trial outcomes and drug development, as seen in the IMvigor 211 trial of atezolizumab (see page 77).

Development of new therapies and rational combinations

There is considerable interest in the outcomes with new drugs, drug classes and combinations, which show great promise and are likely to transform clinical practice after many years with no major improvements. Advances in our understanding of the biology of the complex conditions known as 'bladder cancer' will enable identification of more potential options for treatment. Rational targets for treatment can be identified, lessons learned from other malignancies, and treatments used in other malignancies may be logically evaluated in bladder cancer and existing treatments used more effectively.

The number of potential permutations and combinations of existing and future therapies is daunting, and becomes even more challenging when the various stages of bladder cancer are considered, and the ways in which initial treatment selection may affect subsequent sequencing of treatments. For example, if high-risk non-muscle-invasive disease relapses after systemic immunotherapy, should the patient then receive similar therapy for metastatic disease? If so, when? Would treatment with radiation or chemotherapy modify the probability of a subsequent response to such therapy? Can the initial therapy be modified in some way, such as use in combination with radiation or another ablative technique to prime the immune system so that subsequent immunotherapy is more effective? These and similar questions are hot topics at present, and many clinical trials are planned or underway.

Clinical research must be based on understanding of the clinical imperative to provide benefit to the patient throughout their entire treatment journey, rather than traditional drug development strategies, and it is insufficient to show activity or benefit from one treatment at one stage of the disease. We must understand how and when such treatments should be integrated into the overall treatment course in order to achieve best outcomes for our patients.

The collection of data and samples for future research is also important. Enormous amounts of data are collected as part of routine clinical care but are not available for research or data linkage. For example, clinical samples used for diagnostic purposes are not made available for research. Our patients expect that this sort of work is being done and are often surprised to find it is not. One simple approach would be an opt-in process whereby patients consent to clinical information collected in the context of routine care, and tissue samples surplus to diagnostic requirements, being made available for future research.

Better involvement of palliative and supportive care

Most of the progress in bladder cancer management in the last 20 years has been in supportive care. This relates to improvement in quality of life through better control of symptoms, reduction in treatment-related toxicity, improved management of comorbidities and involvement of other disciplines such as exercise physiology, where improvements in cancer-specific outcomes can also be shown. There is a risk that quality of life is sacrificed by favoring treatments that have good efficacy but might be toxic. Whilst this is understandable, our patients often tell us that quality of life is more important than extending survival.[9] It is important to recognize this, and to remember when considering the choice of treatment in the setting of incurable cancer, that improvement, or at least maintenance, of quality of life and functioning is a paramount objective. It is heartening to see this growing emphasis on patient-reported outcomes. A further benefit from this approach is the focus on reducing and managing the toxicities of treatment, with consequent improvements in response (and potentially cure) rates as well.

Future developments in this area are likely to include:
- improved identification and appropriate streaming of patients through the healthcare system, and management of treatment side-effects[10]
- incorporation of complementary therapies that have been shown to be beneficial in other cancers, such as exercise programs[11]
- improved patient education and empowerment, to ensure toxicities of treatment and complications of the disease are managed appropriately.

Key points – future trends

- Public health preventative measures are likely to have the greatest influence on bladder cancer outcomes globally.
- Earlier diagnosis will shift the pattern of disease towards more favorable stage and grade cancers.
- Outcomes in advanced disease are likely to improve through the uptake of new therapies, including immunotherapy, as well as better application of existing evidence and treatments.
- Improved biological characterization of tumors may point towards more appropriate and patient-specific treatments, including those aimed at specific molecular targets.
- Multidisciplinary management and extended supportive and palliative care measures will increasingly be adopted and improve cancer outcomes and quality of life.

Key references

1. Public Health England. *Adult smoking habits in the UK: 2016.* 2017. www.ons.gov.uk/peoplepopulationandcommunity/healthandsocialcare/healthandlifeexpectancies/bulletins/adultsmokinghabitsingreatbritain/2016#main-points. Last accessed 30 January 2018.

2. Khaled H. Schistosomiasis and cancer in Egypt: review. *J Adv Res* 2013;4:461–6.

3. Stenzl A, Hennenlotter J, Schilling D. Can we still afford bladder cancer? *Curr Opin Urol* 2008;18:488–92.

4. We Care. *Raising awareness of bladder cancer.* 2017. wecarecampaign.org/#about-we-care. Last accessed 30 January 2018.

5. Lerner SP, Goh A. Novel endoscopic diagnosis for bladder cancer. *Cancer* 2015;121:169–78.

6. Hayne D, Stockler M, McCombie SP et al. BCG + Mitomycin trial for high-risk non-muscle-invasive bladder cancer: progress report and lessons learned. *BJU Int* 2017;119(Suppl 5):55–7.

7. Gschwend J, Heck M, Lehmann J et al. Limited versus extended pelvic lymphadenectomy in patients with bladder cancer undergoing radical cystectomy: Survival results from a prospective, randomized trial (LEA AUO AB 25/02). *J Clin Oncol* 2016;34(Suppl 15):abst 4503.

8. Lerner S, Tangen C, Koppie T et al. MP65-02 A phase III surgical trial to evaluate the benefit of a standard versus an extended pelvic lymphadenectomy performed at time of radical cystectomy for muscle invasive urothelial cancer: SWOG S1011 (nct #01224665). *J Urol* 2015;193:e807.

9. Dilla T, Lizan L, Paz S et al. Do new cancer drugs offer good value for money? The perspectives of oncologists, health care policy makers, patients, and the general population. *Patient Pref Adher* 2016;10:1–7.

10. Basch E, Deal AM, Dueck AC et al. Overall survival results of a trial assessing patient-reported outcomes for symptom monitoring during routine cancer treatment. *JAMA* 2017;318:197–8.

11. Cormie P, Zopf EM, Zhang X, Schmitz KH. The impact of exercise on cancer mortality, recurrence, and treatment-related adverse effects. *Epidemiol Rev* 2017;39:1–92.

Useful resources

UK

Action Bladder Cancer UK
Tel: +44 (0)30 0302 0085
info@actionbladdercanceruk.org
actionbladdercanceruk.org/

Cancer Research UK
cancerresearchuk.org/about-cancer/
bladder-cancer

Continence Foundation
info@continence-foundation.org.uk
www.continence-foundation.org.uk

Fight Bladder Cancer
Tel: +44 (0)184 4351 621
info@fightbladdercancer.co.uk
fightbladdercancer.co.uk

UAGBI Urostomy Association
www.uagbi.org

We Care Campaign (Raising Awareness of Bladder Cancer)
wecarecampaign.org

USA

Bladder Cancer Advocacy Network
Tel: +1 301 215 9099
Toll-free: 888 901 BCAN
info@bcan.org
www.bcan.org

National Institutes of Health
Patient information: cancer.gov/types/bladder

Health professional information:
cancer.gov/types/bladder/hp

Oncolink
www.oncolink.org/cancers/urinary-tract/bladder-cancer

International

Bladder Cancer Australia Charity Foundation
contact@bladdercancer.org.au
www.bladdercancer.org.au

Bladder Cancer Canada
Tel: +1 866 674 8889
Info@bladdercancercanada.org
bladdercancercanada.org/en/

Cancer Council Australia
cancer.org.au/about-cancer/types-of-cancer/bladder-cancer.html

Cancer Index
www.cancerindex.org/clinks3d.htm

eviQ
www.eviq.org.au/ (free access; login required)

Index

93

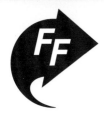

Fast Facts – the ultimate medical handbook series covers over 70 topics, including:

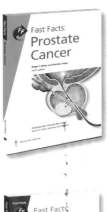

Fast Facts:
Prostate Cancer

Roger S Kirby and Manish I Patel

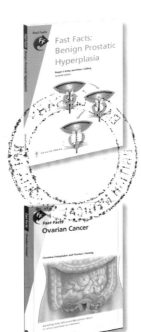

Fast Facts:
Benign Prostatic Hyperplasia

Roger S Kirby and Peter J Gilling
Seventh edition

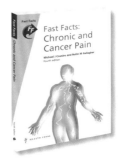

Fast Facts:
Chronic and Cancer Pain

Michael J Cousins and Rollin M Gallagher
Fourth edition

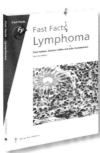

Fast Facts
Lymphoma

Chris Hatton, Graham Collins and John Sweetenham
Second edition

Fast Facts
Ovarian Cancer

Christina Fotopoulou and Thomas J Herzog

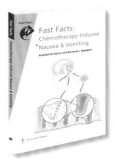

Fast Facts:
Chemotherapy-Induced Nausea & Vomiting

Rudolph M Navari and Bernardo L Rapoport

FastTest

You've read the book ... now test yourself with key questions from the authors

- Go to the FastTest for this title
  FREE at **fastfacts.com**

- Approximate time **10 minutes**

- For best retention of the key issues, try taking the
  FastTest before and after reading